HORMONES AND EVOLUTION

Modern Biology

General Editor

J. E. Webb, Ph.D., D.Sc.
Professor of Zoology
Westfield College, University of London

HORMONES AND EVOLUTION
E. J. W. Barrington M.A., D.Sc.

SPIDERS AND OTHER ARACHNIDS
Theodore Savory M.A., F.Z.S.

ENERGY, LIFE AND ANIMAL ORGANISATION
J. A. Riegel, Ph.D.

HORMONES
AND
EVOLUTION

E. J. W. BARRINGTON, M.A., D.Sc.

Professor of Zoology
University of Nottingham

 THE ENGLISH UNIVERSITIES PRESS LTD

102 NEWGATE STREET · LONDON · EC1

First printed 1964

Printed in Great Britain for the English Universities Press Ltd
by Richard Clay and Company, Ltd, Bungay, Suffolk

Editor's Foreword

THE Modern Biology series is intended to provide the background knowledge to botany and zoology that the upper forms in schools and students in their early years at university need but are unlikely to find in the general textbooks. Each book will give a short authoritative account of an important aspect, a general topic or a new development in biology clearly presented in an extended essay form by an established teacher or research worker in his own field of study.

Scientific matter usually makes heavy demands on the powers of concentration of the reader. Complicated facts and theories are inherently difficult to express in everyday language and frequently hard to understand. Nevertheless much can be done to ease the burden, not only through clear exposition both in text and illustration, but also in the layout and typography of a book.

In *Hormones and Evolution*, Professor Barrington has told a story full of interest and significance so clear that I confidently believe it will convey to all who follow him through these pages the same enthusiasm he undoubtedly feels for his own subject. For my part, as editor, I have done what I can in planning the form of this book to ensure that there is no block to understanding arising from sheer physical difficulty of reading. For instance, the type face and the length and spacing of the lines is such that the book can be read with ease by any normally sighted person even on the top of a bus!

This is, perhaps, an experiment in popularization, but not through the over-simplification of ideas and the avoidance of technicalities which inevitably leads to loss of accuracy. The books in this series are intended to be read as one would read a novel—from cover to cover. There is something in them for all who care to do so. For the student it is hoped they will at once provide examples of the art of the essay in science and a new outlook on biology which will encourage wider reading.

J. E. WEBB

Westfield College
1 August 1963

Preface

THIS book has grown out of three lectures that were given by invitation to the Zoology Departments of the University of London in the autumn of 1961. At that time my intention was to look at some of the problems of comparative endocrinology through the eyes of a zoologist, interested (as which of us is not?) in the origin of animal organization and in the history of its perpetually fascinating adaptations. My intention remains the same, but I have now been able to deploy my arguments in greater detail and with a wider range of examples. In doing so, however, I have become even more conscious of a major difficulty.

The morphologist's interpretation of the evolution of animal structure, and the systematist's interpretation of phylogenetic relationships, rest upon solid foundations laid by generations of workers who devoted themselves to the study of a wide range of species. No such foundation exists for the comparative endocrinologist, nor, indeed, is it easy to find in any branch of comparative physiology. Too few species have as yet been studied, and often the information obtained from these is all too limited. At this stage, then, conclusions must be regarded as very tentative, designed to facilitate the further development of hypotheses and the devising of ways of testing them.

I emphasize this point now in order to avoid having to make repeated and tedious references to it in the text. But it is made only as a warning, and in no sense as an apology, for the reception accorded to my lectures, and to a shortened account of them that appeared in *Experientia*, has encouraged me to suppose that readers will welcome the opportunity of being introduced to a lively branch of biology that is in such an early stage of its own evolution. Those who wish to explore the subject further are recommended to consult some of the books listed on page 147.

I am indebted to Professor J. E. Webb for inviting me to prepare this work, and for his thorough reading of the typescript, and also to my publishers for transforming it so carefully and swiftly into a book. My thanks for the use of copyright illustrations are due to the authors and editors of the works and journals mentioned in the legends, and to the following:

Academic Press, Inc., New York; George Allen and Unwin Ltd., London; Edward Arnold (Publishers) Ltd., London; Birkhäuser Verlag Basel; British Council, medical department; Cambridge University Press; Clarendon Press, Oxford; Company of Biologists Ltd.; Council of the Marine Biological Association of the United Kingdom; English Universities Press Ltd., London; Journal of Physiology; Walter de Gruyter & Co., Berlin; J. P. Lippincott Co., Philadelphia, Pa; Lea & Febiger, Philadelphia, Pa.—Publisher; Macmillan & Co., Ltd., London; Masson & Cie, Paris; Royal Society of Edinburgh; John Wiley & Sons, Inc., New York; Wistar Institute; Zoological Society of London.

E. J. W. BARRINGTON

Contents

1 Evolution and the Endocrine Glands

'Yes; but why didn't it come before?' asked Mrs. Boffin. This draft on Mr. Boffin's philosophy could only be met by that gentleman with the remark that everything that is at all, must begin at some time.
Charles Dickens: *Our Mutual Friend*

Life and Chemical Co-ordination

ENDOCRINE glands and their hormones are a reminder that life is a highly improbable state of matter, dependent for its maintenance upon the success with which highly complex and sensitive chemical systems can continue their activities in a world that is fundamentally hostile to them. This success can only be achieved if the constituent parts of those systems are harmoniously integrated and if the systems are continuously regulated in response to changing conditions within themselves and in the external environment. The progress of organic evolution has therefore depended upon the establishment of co-ordinating mechanisms, and the importance of the chemical agents known as hormones lies in the contributions that they have made to this fundamental requirement of life.

The credit for having been the first to provide an experimental demonstration of hormonal action is commonly given to Berthold for his observations on domestic capons. These are male birds that have been castrated, and one consequence of the operation is that they lack the well-developed comb and wattle of animals not operated upon.   Berthold showed in 1849 that they would develop normal sexual characteristics and behaviour if testes were transplanted into their abdominal cavities, and we now know that this is because vertebrate testes, in addition to producing sperm, act also as endocrine glands.   The function of these is to discharge a secretion that regulates sexual development, so that injection of this secretion, or of substances related to it (p. 52), produces the same effect as implantation of the organs themselves (Fig. 1).

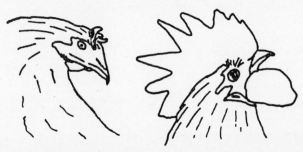

Fig. 1.   *Left*, the head of a capon.   *Right*, the head of the same animal after 22 daily injections of an androgen (androsterone).   After Parkes, 1935, *Biochem. J.*, 29, 1422, from Barrington, 1963, *Introduction to General and Comparative Endocrinology* (Oxford: Clarendon Press).

However, it took time for the true significance of Berthold's work to be fully appreciated, and the term endocrine was not introduced into biological science until nearly the end of the century.   Even then its first application was not to the glandular tissue of the testes, but to the islets of Langerhans in the pancreas (Fig. 2).   Laguesse, in introducing it, was giving expression to the idea that these groups of cells, clearly distinguishable from those containing the digestive enzymes, might be producing a secretion that was discharged internally into the blood stream (*endon*, within; *krinein*, to separate), instead of being released, like the exocrine secretion of digestive enzymes, through an external duct (*exo*, outwards).   This idea was in fact, very well founded, but it was not finally established as correct until the hormone insulin (p. 21) was discovered over twenty years later.

As for the term hormone itself, this was introduced in 1902 by Bayliss and Starling as a result of their fundamentally important investigations into the mechanism by which the discharge of the pancreatic enzymes was regulated in mammals. They had concluded that the entry into the duodenum of the acid contents of the

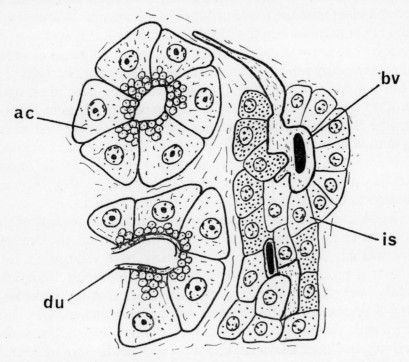

Fig. 2. Exocrine and endocrine components of the pancreas of a mammal. *ac.*, acinus, formed of a group of exocrine cells with large zymogen granules; *bv.*, blood vessel; *du.*, ductule, leading from an acinus; *is.*, islet of Langerhans, formed of a group of endocrine cells with small granules.

stomach stimulated the intestinal wall to release into the blood stream a substance that they called secretin. This substance, they believed, was carried to the pancreas, where it directly stimulated that organ to release its exocrine secretion, with the result that the pancreatic enzymes arrived in the duodenum at just the right time to act upon the food material, and thus to continue the digestive processes that had been initiated in the stomach (Fig. 8, p. 20).

This idea of chemical co-ordination constituted an important new principle that was likely to have wider applications, and they therefore suggested that substances acting in the manner of secretin might be called hormones, a term derived from the Greek *hormaein*, meaning to arouse or to stimulate.

A hormone can thus be defined as a substance that is manufactured in a particular tissue or organ of the animal concerned and that is then released into the blood stream so that it is able to exert specific regulatory effects elsewhere in the body, its points of action being commonly referred to as its target cells or target organs.   It is to be noted that the idea of a hormone being dependent upon transport in the blood stream is an important element in this classical definition, although it is not included in the original meaning of the Greek root.   Equally important is the fact that hormones contribute nothing either to the structural elements of the organs that they regulate or to their energy supplies, so that they are required to be produced in only very minute amounts.

The idea of chemical interactions between different parts of the body was by no means new at the time when Bayliss and Starling were working, although they could justly have claimed to have given it a profoundly new significance.   Quite apart from Berthold's work, it had already been established that myxoedema, a form of premature senile decay in adult human beings, was associated with the presence of a defective thyroid gland, and this condition had been alleviated in a most spectacular way by feeding thyroid-gland preparations to a patient.   Then again, to take only one other example, it had been shown by Oliver and Schäfer in 1895 that the injection into experimental mammals of extracts of the adrenal gland could affect certain muscular tissues and produce a remarkable rise in blood pressure.

Such results, however, seemed at the time to be of somewhat limited significance, for they appeared to demonstrate only the effects of some pathological condition in an organ, or the pharmacological properties of its extracts, and a full appreciation of their importance did not, therefore, develop until later.   The wider perspective opened up by Bayliss and Starling's discovery was a crucial factor in this, and it is interesting for zoologists to reflect that another significant advance was the demonstration of the consequences of feeding thyroid-gland material to frog tadpoles. This, as Gudernatsch first showed in 1912, evokes a premature metamorphosis, a result that indicates very clearly how the secretion of a single organ may have the most profound influence upon the co-ordinated growth and development of the whole animal.

The concept of hormones, then, did not emerge fully fledged. From its first formulation it had to be developed and extended, and we shall see that this remains true even today. Nevertheless, the form in which we have stated it here, and which we may think of as the classical form of the concept, remains a valuable starting point for a discussion of the evolutionary history of these agents, and we can conveniently develop our argument from it.

Hormones, Vitamins, and Evolution

Since chemical co-ordination is such a fundamental feature of animal organization, it is not surprising to find that the existence of endocrine glands is widespread throughout the animal kingdom. The situation is best understood, however, in vertebrates, the endocrine system of which is outlined in diagrammatic form in Fig. 3. No zoologist who names the glands shown in that illustration would doubt that the possession of these organs serves in itself to distinguish vertebrates from all other groups of animals. It is true that the endocrine glands of the lower members of the group may sometimes differ in their arrangement and appearance from those of mammals, but such differences are commonly of a minor character, and a set of histological preparations of these organs presents an appearance entirely characteristic of the vertebrates, irrespective of the evolutionary status of the animal from which they are selected.

Most zoologists would probably also feel that the same might be said of the secretory products of these glands (Table 1), for to enumerate them—growth hormone, oxytocin, testosterone, cortisone, adrenaline, and others that we shall refer to later—is to suggest a complex of substances possessed by no other group of the animal kingdom. Nevertheless, we cannot feel that the unique character of this endocrine complex is quite so readily demonstrable at the chemical level as it seems to be at the histological and

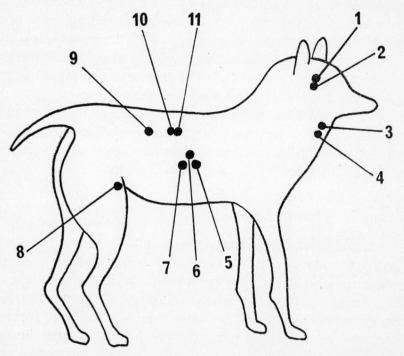

Fig. 3. Distribution of major components of the endocrine system of a mammal. *1*, hypothalamus; *2*, adenohypophysis; *3*, thyroid gland; *4*, parathyroid gland; *5*, stomach; *6*, pancreas; *7*, intestine; *8*, testis (in male); *9*, ovary (in female); *10*, adrenocortical tissue, and *11*, chromaffin tissue, these two forming the adrenal gland.

morphological ones. The distribution of adrenaline, for example, is certainly not restricted to the vertebrates (p. 67), and we still know far too little of the secretions of invertebrate animals to be able to say with certainty whether or not any particular product of vertebrates is restricted to the latter, although in some instances the evidence for such restriction is very strong indeed. However, what we can say with some assurance is that nowhere else in the animal kingdom do we find this same complete equipment of hor-

SOURCE	HORMONE	CHEMICAL NATURE
Hypothalamus	Oxytocin	Polypeptide
	Vasopressin	Polypeptide
Adenohypophysis		
Pars distalis	Growth hormone	Protein
	Thyrotropin	Glycoprotein
	Corticotropin	Polypeptide
	Follicle-stimulating hormone	Glycoprotein (sheep)
	Interstitial cell-stimulating hormone	Mucoprotein (sheep)
	Prolactin (luteotropin)	Protein
Pars intermedia	Melanocyte-stimulating hormone	Polypeptide
Thyroid	3,5,3′-Tri-iodothyronine	Iodinated amino acid
	Thyroxine	Iodinated amino acid
Parathyroid	Parathormone	Protein
Stomach	Gastrin	?
Pancreas	Insulin	Protein
	Glucagon	Polypeptide
Intestine	Secretin	Polypeptide
	Pancreozymin	?
	Cholecystokinin	?
Testis	Testosterone	Steroid
Ovary	Oestradiol	Steroid
Adrenocortical tissue	Cortisol (hydrocortisone)	Steroid
	Corticosterone	Steroid
	Aldosterone	Steroid
Chromaffin tissue	Adrenaline	Catecholamine
	Noradrenaline	Catecholamine

Table 1

Some Hormones of Mammals

Note that the larger polypeptide molecules (e.g. corticotropin, glucagon) might equally well be termed small protein molecules. Further references to the properties of many of these hormones will be found in the text (cf. Fig. 3, p. 6).

mones working together in the closely integrated way that characterizes the co-ordinating machinery of vertebrates. This amounts to asserting that the evolution of that group has involved the establishment not only of such familiar structures as gill slits, notochord, and hollow dorsal nervous system but also of a particular and unique pattern in the endocrine system. In other words, that system is in its total organization a novelty, and its existence has to be explained as a result of the appearance of something new, and not merely as an inheritance from remote ancestors.

The implications of this situation can be illustrated by drawing a comparison with certain of the vitamins, for these are substances that resemble hormones in so far as they are required in only minute amounts for the maintenance of normal activity, without themselves contributing either energy or structural elements to the body. There is an important difference, however, in that animals are unable to achieve the complete synthesis of their own vitamin requirements. They must therefore look to their food to supply either the vitamins themselves or, in certain cases, specific precursor substances called provitamins that can be readily transformed into them. Should animals fail to obtain this supply, they may die, or develop deficiency diseases, each of which is specifically characteristic of the lack of a particular vitamin.

Some vitamins seem to be a requirement for all forms of life, ranging from micro-organisms to the higher plants and animals, and an example is provided by thiamine (vitamin B_1), the absence of which causes beri-beri in man and polyneuritis in the pigeon and rat. Its importance depends upon the fact that the release of energy within the cell involves certain fundamental metabolic pathways that seem to have been established at a very early stage in evolution, and to have become, in consequence, a common inheritance of all living organisms. An example of this is seen in the release of energy from glucose, a common pathway for which involves the transformation of that substance to pyruvic acid. The carboxyl group of the latter is next removed by oxidative decarboxylation, and the remaining acetyl group can then be metabolized by the complex of enzymes that forms the Krebs, or citric acid, cycle. In this sequence of events the decarboxylation of pyruvic acid is mediated by the enzyme carboxylase, and the explanation of the importance of thiamine is that carboxylase can function only in association with a co-enzyme called cocarboxylase, a substance that proves to be the pyrophosphate of thiamine. Thus, the universal need for this vitamin is seen to be a consequence of its involvement as an obligatory component of a fundamental metabolic pathway in the cell.

The thiamine molecule is formed of a pyrimidine and a thiazole component (Fig. 4), and many micro-organisms can synthesize both of these for themselves, so that they do not need to obtain the molecule from external sources. Other micro-organisms, however, can synthesize only one component, while still others can synthesize neither, and this latter position is the one in which metazoan

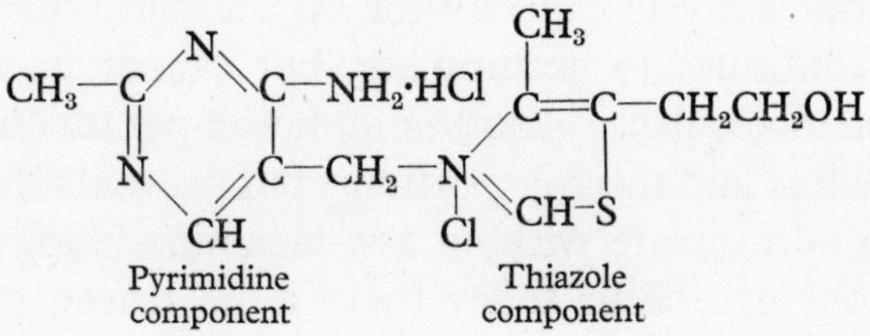

Pyrimidine component   Thiazole component

Fig. 4. Molecular structure of thiamine (vitamin B_1) chloride hydrochloride.

animals also find themselves. They, therefore, must obtain their thiamine from their food (unless, as happens in many insects and mammals, it is synthesized for them by micro-organisms in their alimentary tract), and it is for them that thiamine is a vitamin, a molecule that is essential for their life, but which they are unable to produce for themselves.

Certain other vitamins of the B group have a status essentially similar to that of thiamine, and it may well be asked, when such substances are so widely needed and for such essential functions, why so many organisms have to meet their requirements from external sources of supply. We cannot feel sure of the answer to this question, but a widely favoured explanation is that initially these materials were part of the organized system of evolving proto-plasm. Then, it is suggested, genetic mutations (p. 14) led to the loss of the capacity for synthesizing one or other of them, an event that still happens today in laboratory cultures of the mould *Neurospora*.

Neurospora can normally synthesize its requirement of thiamine; indeed, it can be grown in the laboratory on a medium containing no more than sugar, biotin (one of the B vitamins), and inorganic salts.   If, however, it is exposed to chemicals such as mustard oil or formaldehyde, which have the capacity for accelerating its normal rate of genetic mutation, various mutant strains are obtained that require additional metabolites to be added to the medium if these strains are to grow at a normal rate.   This is taken to mean that each such strain has lost, by virtue of a specific mutation, the power of synthesizing a particular substance, so that this substance has now to be added from an external source.   One mutation, for example, eliminates the capacity for synthesizing thiazole, so that pyrimidine continues to accumulate, but cannot be incorporated into thiamine molecules.   Another mutation permits the formation of the pyrimidine and thiazole portions, but prevents their coupling, so that both accumulate without any thiamine being formed.   If such mutations can occur today there is no reason to doubt that they must have occurred in the past, and at the earliest stages of evolution.   Moreover, it may be assumed that they occurred in animals as well as in plants, but that the former were able to survive such loss because the substance that they were no longer able to synthesize was readily obtainable from plants.   These deficiencies could therefore have remained as an acceptable and permanent element of the biochemical organization of the animal kingdom.

On this view the dependence of living organisms upon these B vitamins is interpreted as a consequence of regressive evolution, which has involved the loss of the capacity for synthesizing certain clearly defined agents of cell metabolism.   If this is so, it follows that the evolutionary history of such vitamins must have been very different from that of animal hormones, for, although we still know little of how the latter function at the cellular level, we certainly gain the impression that they are often needed not to maintain an animal's life, but rather to regulate, and perhaps to facilitate, some aspect or other of its activity.   This implies that they must have been introduced relatively late into living systems that were already fully functional; they must, therefore, be the result of the evolution of new synthetic capacities, and from this point of view they differ fundamentally from the B vitamins that we have discussed.

However, the view that the dependence of organisms upon certain B vitamins is a result of the loss of synthetic capacities is not applicable to all vitamins, for some of these present a situation much more closely akin to that of the hormones, and we may very well look to them to see whether they can provide any guide to the possible history of the latter. An example of this is vitamin A, a substance that is known in two closely related forms, vitamin A_1 and vitamin A_2, the latter, with two double bonds in its ring, being particularly characteristic of freshwater fish. Vitamin A is an essential requirement of mammals, lack of it resulting in lesions of the mucous membranes, disturbance of growth, and diminished resistance to infection; in addition, it plays an important part in the cycle of photochemical pigments in the retina of the eye. Its significance in lower vertebrates is less clear, but it is certainly found in their retinae, and the fact that these animals contain stores of it elsewhere in the body, and particularly in the liver, suggests that in them, as in mammals, it may have more generalized functions additional to its retinal one.

In contrast to the widespread need for the B vitamins, however, there is no conclusive evidence that vitamin A is an essential requirement for the maintenance of the life of any invertebrate animal, although locusts are said to require either this substance or carotene (see below). It is, therefore, all the more interesting from our present point of view to find that its presence in vertebrates is certainly not its first or only appearance in the animal kingdom, for it occurs also, as vitamin A_1, in the eyes of crustaceans and cephalopods, although it is doubtful whether it has any function in these animals other than a visual one.

A further fact of importance for our analysis is that although the vitamin A molecules are characteristically animal products, they are derived from certain carotenoid pigments, a group of substances that are widely distributed in both the plant and the animal kingdoms (Fig. 5). The vitamin-forming members of this group, which can be regarded as provitamins, have always to be obtained from plant sources, since animals are incapable of synthesizing them; once possessed of them however, crustaceans as well as vertebrates are apparently able to transform them into vitamin A.

The full significance of this wide distribution of carotenoids remains somewhat obscure, although they are thought to protect the cells of plants from the harmful effects of the light that is absorbed

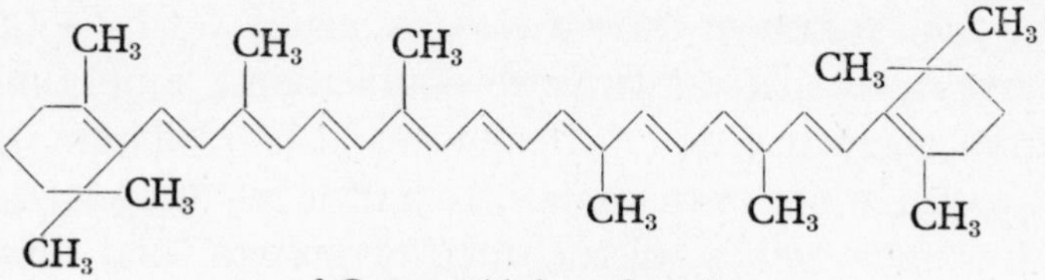

β-Carotene (skeleton formula)

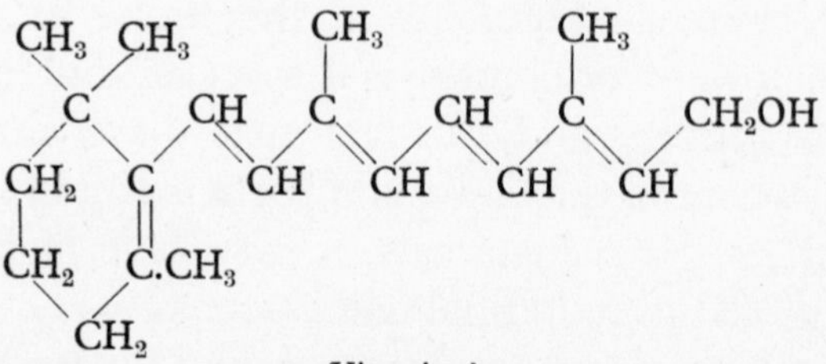

Vitamin A$_1$

Fig. 5. Molecular structure of β-carotene and vitamin A$_1$. From Walsh, 1961, *An Introduction to Biochemistry* (London: English Univ. Press).

by chlorophyll, and they seem to be widely employed in photoreceptor systems from micro-organisms upwards, as, for example, in the eye-spot of flagellate Protozoa. In any case, it is clear that the development of vitamin A in the eyes of crustaceans, cephalopods, and vertebrates can be viewed as a result of a further evolution of a type of molecule that was already widely distributed in nature. Moreover, the vitamin is found in invertebrates exclusively in the form of vitamin A$_1$, so that the appearance of vitamin A$_2$ in freshwater fish is another illustration of such evolution. The extension of the activity of the vitamin beyond the field of visual function in mammals (and probably in other vertebrates also) indicates that the sphere of action of this substance has been enlarged during vertebrate evolution. This enlargement, it will be observed, has apparently involved no further change in the molecule itself, which suggests that it must be due to the cells concerned having developed a capacity for responding to it in a specialized way. This is a concept of considerable potential interest, and we shall have occasion to refer to it more than once when we pass to consider the contribution that has apparently been made to the evolution of endocrine systems by the specialization of target cells.

The several forms of vitamin D, to take one other example (Fig. 6), present a situation somewhat similar to that of vitamin A,

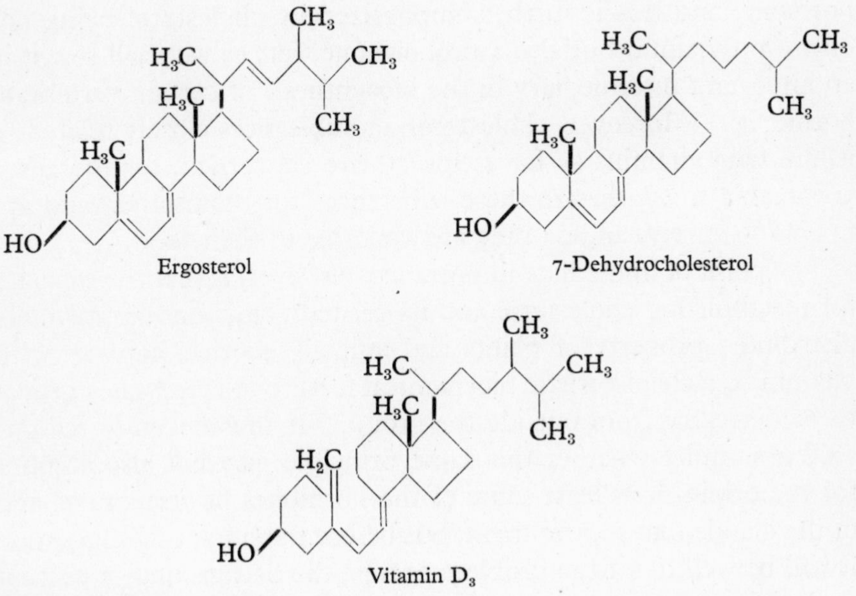

Fig. 6. Molecular structure of vitamin D_3 and related compounds (cf. Fig. 21, p. 45).

for this vitamin, too, is a characteristically vertebrate requirement, being essential in mammals for the maintenance of the normal metabolism of calcium and phosphorus. It is related chemically to the sterols, of which we shall have much to say later, and it can be formed by the ultraviolet irradiation of ergosterol (forming vitamin D_2) or, in the animal body, of 7-dehydrocholesterol (forming vitamin D_3), so that these two sterols (Fig. 6) are pro-vitamins for vitamin D, just as are carotenoids for vitamin A.

There is, however, an important difference, in that 7-dehydro-cholesterol, unlike the carotenoids, can be manufactured by mammals from cholesterol, which itself can be synthesized from acetate (p. 54). In practice, of course, the supply of ultraviolet light may be inadequate for synthesis of the vitamin, so that reliance has to be placed upon dietary sources of the latter, such as fish oils. Nevertheless, the fact that even part of the vitamin D requirement of a mammal can be manufactured within the body goes some way to narrow the distinction between a vitamin and a hormone, and this is further emphasized by cholesterol being not only a provitamin but also a prohormone, for, as we shall see, it is an important intermediary in the biosynthesis of certain vertebrate hormones. Moreover, cholesterol, or substances closely related to it, are true vitamins as far as insects are concerned, for the latter are unable to synthesize these substances for themselves, and are unable to survive unless they are available in their food.

The point of immediate importance, however, is that the capacity for metabolizing cholesterol and its related compounds is a widely distributed property of plants and animals, so that here, as with vitamin A, a characteristic biochemical feature of vertebrates proves to be derivable from outside the group. It thus becomes reasonable to enquire whether this same principle may not also account for the origin of at least some of the hormones of vertebrates and of the glands that secrete them, but before pursuing this suggestion it will be well to set the problem against the background of current evolutionary theory.

This rests primarily upon the concept of evolution as being dependent upon the unique properties of macromolecular strings of deoxyribonucleic acid (DNA), which, situated in the chromosomes, have the capacity both for self-replication and also for the self-variation that we call mutation. The sites of these mutations are called genes, and these, in classical Mendelian theory, have been regarded as particulate units, the transmission of which from parents to offspring constitutes the physical basis of heredity. Recent advances in our knowledge of chromosome structure make it difficult to decide whether these genes are, in fact, sharply delimited from each other, or whether they simply represent regions of the chromosomes with no very definite boundaries. The problem need not concern us here. It will be sufficient to say that these mutations, and the recombinations that they undergo at sexual reproduction, provide the raw material for the action of natural selection. The effect of this action upon a species is to promote the establishment of those variants that confer some adaptive advantage upon a particular population, an advantage that is expressed in an improvement of its chances of survival.

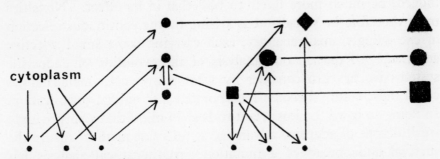

Fig. 7. Diagrammatic representation of the progressive interaction of genes and cytoplasm during development. Starting at the left, part of the cytoplasm of the developing egg reacts with genes (small circles) to produce three substances, two of which interact with each other. At a later stage these substances react with other genes to produce new substances. The central 'square' is a key substance, interacting with genes to form the large 'circle' and transforming the 'diamond' into the 'triangle'. Mutation in one of the first set of three genes may thus have far-reaching effects. After Waddington, 1957, *The Strategy of the Genes* (London: Allen and Unwin).

It is supposed that the immediate effect of a mutation upon a cell is to produce some modification in the biochemical capacities of the latter. Often this must result from the gene concerned having a controlling influence upon an intracellular enzyme system, sometimes, perhaps, because it determines the synthesis of an individual enzyme. The result of this is that the influence of the mutation will become apparent in its effect upon some reaction pattern, affecting, for example, the course of cell differentiation, or the establishment of particular metabolic pathways and their products, with consequences likely to be widely disseminated throughout the organism during the course of its development (Fig. 7). Earlier ideas of each mutation as having a single and sharply definable effect upon a specific character are therefore no longer acceptable; instead, we must think of them as having multiple effects, this being the phenomenon known as pleiotropy.

Partly because of this last consideration, another earlier suggestion, that novelties might arise as the result of a single mutation with a substantial effect, has also been discarded. It is now appreciated that such a change would so disturb established organization that it could rarely, if ever, have any survival value, but would, indeed, be much more likely to be lethal in its effect. Novelties must therefore be visualized as arising by the continuous selection of exceedingly small changes, each carrying some small selective advantage, so that in our analysis of the evolution of endocrine systems we have to consider by what paths such small changes could most readily become incorporated into animal organization. In doing so it will be important to bear in mind that a surprisingly small degree of adaptive advantage is fully adequate to ensure the survival and spread of a mutation. Mathematical analysis has shown, in fact, that a favourable mutation may be expected to become established in a population if its selective advantage is no more than 1%, by which is meant that 101 offspring carrying the mutation will survive for every 100 offspring that survive without it.

It is because of this that the demonstration of the presence in one group of animals of molecules identical with, or closely similar to, the hormonal molecules of another group can often be very illuminating. The two groups concerned may have no close relationship with each other, yet the presence in one of them of even trace quantities of such molecules may suggest ways in which these might have first appeared in the other group, where, perhaps, some special circumstance of biochemical organization may have enabled these molecules to give some slight selective advantage. We have already encountered this possibility in our comparison of vitamins with hormones, which suggested that the synthesis of biologically important substances in vertebrates might sometimes have had its inception in the presence of these or closely related substances in other forms of life, and we shall refer to it again when we are dealing in detail with the molecular structure of hormones.

The Endocrine System of Vertebrates

The possible modes of origin of novel features of animal organization have been outlined by Mayr in the proposition that a new structure or property may be thought of as arising in one or other of three ways. The first possibility is that it may arise from a mutation that initially has an advantage in some quite different direction, the germ of the new feature being some pleiotropic by-product that at first has no selective advantage at all. The second possibility is that it may arise as a result of an intensification of some already existing function, while a third possibility is that it may result from some change of function in an already existing organ.

Of these three possibilities, the first may be the least important, and it will certainly be difficult to establish in any particular case, for it requires the demonstration of a negative. The other two, however, and more particularly the third, are probably of wider significance, and it will be noticed that both of them carry the implication that the appearance of novelty in organization is not necessarily associated with the evolution of an entirely new structure or mechanism. This suggestion has already emerged from our discussion of the vitamins. All three possibilities will be found to provide a helpful basis for our discussion of the evolution of endocrine systems, and we can best form a first impression of their validity by testing them against our present understanding of the history of vertebrate endocrine organs. We can then proceed to extend their application to the problems of the evolution of the hormones themselves.

This evolution has undoubtedly been a very long process. The earliest fossil traces of vertebrates are found as bony fragments in Ordovician deposits, while remains of recognizable animals are well known from the Silurian and Devonian periods, so that the history of the group can be estimated as extending over more than 400 million years. The interpretation of this history, and the establishment of the phylogenetic relationships of the highly diversified forms that have arisen in the course of it, present many problems that we shall not attempt to consider here. It is necessary, however, to keep in mind an outline classification of the vertebrates, so that some estimate can be made of the evolutionary status of the animals that we shall mention. One such outline, omitting many extinct groups, could be as follows, although variants upon this are possible and acceptable:

Phylum Chordata
    Subphylum Hemichordata
      (e.g. *Balanoglossus, Saccoglossus*)
    Subphylum Tunicata (Urochordata)
      (e.g. the sea-squirts, such as *Ciona*)
    Subphylum Cephalochordata
      (e.g. *Branchiostoma* (amphioxus))
    Subphylum Vertebrata (Craniata)
      Grade Agnatha (jawless vertebrates, mostly extinct)
        Class Cyclostomata
          (lampreys and hagfish)
      Grade Gnathostomata (jawed vertebrates)
        Class Placodermi (extinct fish with primitive jaws)
        Class Elasmobranchii
          (dogfish, sharks, rays)
        Class Actinopterygii
          (most living bony fish, including Teleostei such as *Salmo* and *Gasterosteus*)
        Class Crossopterggii
          (the living lung-fish, such as *Protopterus*, and the extinct ancestors of land vertebrates)
        Class Amphibia
        Class Reptilia
        Class Aves
        Class Mammalia

It will be apparent from this scheme that the vertebrates do not constitute an isolated group of the animal kingdom, but are a

Subphylum that forms the major part of a larger group, the Phylum Chordata. The three remaining Subphyla, commonly referred to as the Protochordata, are generally believed to be closely related to the Echinodermata, the group that includes starfish and sea-urchins, and to be widely separated from such familiar inverte-brates as the insects, crustaceans, and molluscs. The systematic position of the Hemichordata is a matter for some dispute, and there are authors who would regard them as invertebrates, although still very close to the chordate line of ancestry. The other two protochordate Subphyla, however, share certain clearly defined vertebrate features, such as the notochord, so that although their surviving members are not direct ancestors of the vertebrates, it is certain that the latter must have been derived from some proto-chordate type of organization. Protochordates, then, represent the stage of evolution at which the foundations of vertebrate mor-phology and physiology were being laid, and we shall therefore have much to say of them in due course, despite the fact that endo-crine organs are not a conspicuous feature of their structure. Even with their help, however, it is not always possible to find visible evidence of the evolutionary history of vertebrate endocrine organs, and in some instances even the very existence of these has to be inferred from their physiological effects, a situation that we can illustrate by a further reference to secretin (Fig. 8). We now know that this is one member of a complex of hormones that are secreted within the alimentary tract and that regulate, in co-operation with the nervous system, the passage of food and the discharge of di-gestive secretions. Secretin is concerned with the release of the fluid part of the pancreatic secretion, and probably also with the secretion of bile by the liver, while pancreozymin, also secreted in the duodenum, and not recognized until recently as being distinct from secretin, regulates the release of the pancreatic enzymes. Other members of the complex are gastrin, secreted by the stomach, and regulating the secretion of the acid component of the gastric juice, and cholecystokinin, secreted in the intestine, and controlling the discharge of bile from the gall bladder. There may be other members, for the system remains in some obscurity, partly because of the technical difficulty of studying it. It is reasonable to suppose, however, that it has evolved as a specialization of the fundamental secretory capacity of the alimentary tract, and that

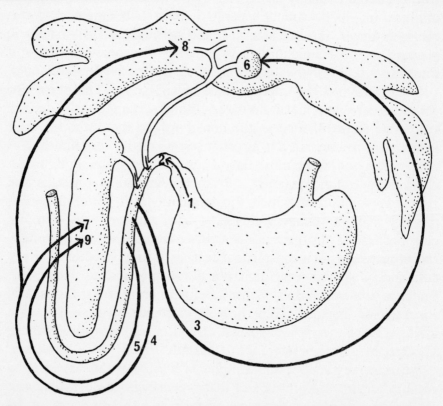

Fig. 8. Some of the endocrine pathways that regulate digestion in a mammal. The passage of gastric contents from the stomach (*1*) into the duodenum (*2*) evokes the release from the latter of three hormones, cholecystokinin (*3*), secretin (*4*), and pancreozymin (*5*). Cholecystokinin evokes contractions of the gall bladder (*6*), secretin stimulates the secretion of fluid from the pancreas (*7*), and of bile from the liver (*8*), while pancreozymin stimulates the secretion of the pancreatic enzymes (*9*). The secretions of the liver and pancreas are thus discharged into the duodenum (*2*) in appropriate quantities at the correct time.

the absence of clearly differentiated endocrine tissue is a consequence of the system having remained at a primitive level of organization.

This is the more probable in that the alimentary tract is also the ultimate source of other hormones, for the pancreas, which grows out from the anterior end of the intestine at an early stage of embryonic development, not only secretes the digestive pancreatic juice but also contains endocrine tissue, the islets of Langerhans (Fig. 2), to which we have already referred. This tissue secretes two substances, the hormone insulin, important as a regulator of metabolic processes, and glucagon, which may also be a metabolic hormone, although its status has still to be fully clarified.

Something of the past history of the pancreas can be deduced from an examination of those very primitive vertebrates, the lampreys, for in them the organ is not morphologically differentiated despite the presence of a well-developed liver. Secretory cells concentrated at the anterior end of the intestine probably represent the exocrine component of that organ at a stage at which its separation from the secretory lining of the intestine has not begun, while the endocrine component is probably represented by groups of cells, called the follicles of Langerhans, that are budded off from the same region of that epithelium, but remain embedded in the submucosa. Thus, although the pancreas appears in higher vertebrates as a morphological novelty, it is clearly possible to interpret it, along the lines of the second possibility outlined above, as a further specialization of the long-standing secretory capacity of the intestinal epithelium.

We must be careful, of course, not to overstate the position by regarding this suggestion as offering a complete explanation why the alimentary epithelium should have begun to secrete hormones in the first instance. Nevertheless, it is possible to see a certain logic in such a development. The digestive epithelium is concerned with the transport of future metabolites from the lumen of the alimentary canal into the blood stream, and it may be that its sensitivity to such substances led some of its cells towards a capacity for responding to the varying amounts of the metabolites in the circulating blood. Such responsiveness might take the form of fluctuations in the discharge by these cells of their own metabolic products, one or more of which could then be adapted into a hormone under the influence of natural selection. This is, of course, a highly theoretical argument, but the principle involved, the evolution of a hormone from a product of cell metabolism, has been plausibly suggested as an explanation of the origin of more than one vertebrate hormone (pp. 25, 60). It may be said to conform broadly with the first of our three possibilities, which was that new features of organization might arise as by-products of existing features.

Two other important endocrine organs arise from the alimentary tract, in this case from the pharynx, and both could be held to illustrate our third possibility, a change of function in an existing organ. One of these is the parathyroid gland, secreting a hormone (parathormone) that is involved in the regulation of calcium and

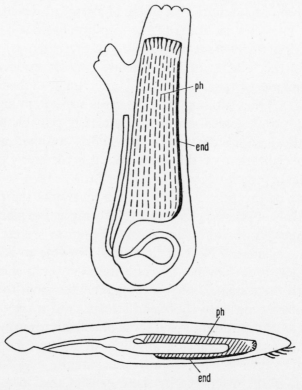

Fig. 9. Diagrams of *Ciona* (*above*, ×⅔) and *Branchiostoma* (*below*, × 2), to show the positions of the endostyle (*end.*) and pharynx (*ph.*). From Barrington, 1962, *Experientia*, **18**, 201–210.

phosphorus metabolism. The parathyroid gland is absent from fish, but it appears in tetrapod embryos as a derivative of the vestigial branchial pouches, so that at this rather crude level of analysis it might be regarded as an example of a change of function in an already existing tissue. Unfortunately, too little is known about this particular evolutionary problem to justify further discussion of it here, but we have much more complete information regarding the other pharyngeal derivative, the thyroid gland.

Important clues to the history of this gland are provided by the

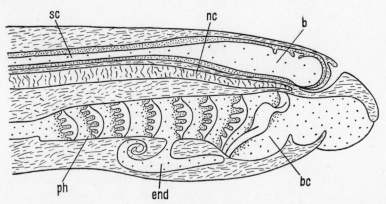

Fig. 10. Vertical longitudinal section (diagrammatic) through the anterior end of the ammocoete larva of the lamprey. *b.*, brain; *bc.*, buccal cavity; *end.*, endostyle; *nc.*, notochord; *ph.*, pharynx; *sc.*, spinal cord. From Barrington, 1962, *Experientia*, **18**, 201–210.

tunicates and amphioxus (Fig. 9), for in the floor of the pharynx of these animals there is a secretory and ciliated groove, the endostyle, which plays a leading part in the ciliary feeding that is so characteristic of protochordates. This organ persists, although in a modified form, in the larva of the lamprey (Fig. 10), but at metamorphosis it in part disappears and in part gives rise to the thyroid gland. This has long been regarded as a classical example of the evolution of an endocrine organ by the transformation of function in an already existing organ, but at the level of such embryological and anatomical analysis we are clearly unable to secure a complete understanding of the course of events. We must ask, for example, whether the change of function is foreshadowed in any way in the

B

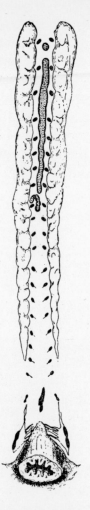

Fig. 11. Arrangement of chromaffin tissue (double row of black bodies) and adrenocortical tissue (stippled) in the dogfish *Mustelus canis*. The kidneys have been turned outwards to uncover these structures; the adrenocortical tissue and the more caudal chromaffin bodies are within the kidneys, the more anterior chromaffin bodies are dorsal to them. From Hartman and Brownell, 1949, *The Adrenal Gland* (Philadelphia, Pa.: Lea and Febiger).

protochordates of the present day, and whether it is possible to determine the circumstances in which the thyroid hormones were first synthesized by the chordates. These questions take us directly into the field of biochemical evolution, and we shall return to them later.

The mesoderm of the vertebrate embryo is another important source of endocrine glands, for the interstitial tissue of the gonads and the adrenocortical tissue both develop from it. We shall be discussing later the steroid hormones that are secreted by these tissues (and also, to some extent, by the mammalian placenta), and it will be sufficient now to say that their functions extend into the regulation of the control of the water and salt-electrolyte content of the body fluids, and the maintenance of reproductive activity.

Accounts of the development of the gonads and adrenocortical tissue are not always quite consistent, but the regions of the meso-derm that are particularly concerned are the coelomic epithelium and the nephrotomes that give rise to the mesonephric kidney tubules. Willmer has suggested that the association of these regions with the regulation of the body fluids and of reproduction may be a result of the involvement of the coelom and its contained fluid in excretory and reproductive processes. The coelomoducts, which place the coelom in communication with the external en-vironment, serve in many animals for the passage of excretory products and germ cells, so that it is possible to imagine that when vertebrates were first evolving some of the cells of those ducts might have come to respond to fluctuations in excretory and repro-ductive activities. Hormones might then have evolved out of their metabolic products, much as we have suggested in connexion with the evolution of the islets of Langerhans. As with the thyroid gland, however, purely morphological considerations have their limitations, so that we shall have to look to the molecular structure of the hormones concerned for further clues to their origin.

In elasmobranch fish the adrenocortical tissue (Fig. 11) is scattered widely along the dorsal wall of the coelom and in the kidney, but in higher forms it becomes more compact, and eventu-ally constitutes in mammals the outer layer, or cortex, of the adrenal gland (Fig. 12); it is, of course, from this final stage in its morphological history that it takes its name. There is also present in fish another scattered tissue, the chromaffin tissue (Fig. 11), so called because granules in its cells develop a yellow-brown colour on being treated with certain reagents such as potassium dichro-mate. This tissue also becomes more compact in higher forms, and enters into increasingly close association with the adrenocortical tissue, eventually becoming established in mammals as the central medulla of the adrenal gland. It is surprising, but nevertheless a useful reminder of our ignorance of much that has conditioned the evolution of endocrine systems, that as yet we have no satisfactory explanation of the functional significance of this association, although the facts have long been familiar to students of comparative anatomy.

The functional relationships of the chromaffin tissue are of par-

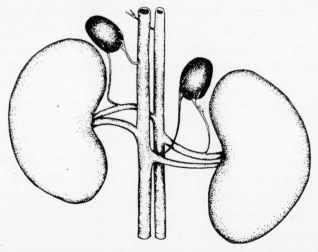

Fig. 12. The adrenal glands (*dark*) and kidneys (*light*) in the white-footed mouse, *Peromyscus leucopus noveboracensis*. From Hartman and Brownell, 1949, *The Adrenal Gland* (Philadelphia, Pa.: Lea and Febiger).

ticular interest. Its secretion consists of adrenaline and the closely similar noradrenaline (Fig. 28, p. 68), two hormones having a variety of effects that, as far as mammals are concerned, can be summed up as being particularly concerned with facilitating the response of the animal to sudden demands made upon it at moments of crisis and strain. The chromaffin tissue is formed of cells that migrate out of the developing sympathetic ganglia, and is further linked with the nervous system by virtue of the fact that noradrenaline is secreted at the nerve endings of the post-ganglionic nerve fibres of the sympathetic system. Noradrenaline, and also acetylcholine, which is secreted at many other nerve endings in vertebrates, are known as chemical transmitter substances, the function of these being to bridge the gap, or synapse, between one nerve fibre and another, or to link the nerve fibres with the effector cells that they innervate. The nerve impulse itself cannot pass across the gaps separating these structures, but its arrival at the ending of a nerve fibre results in the release of a minute quantity of one of these transmitter substances, and it is this that activates the adjacent nerve fibre, or the effector cell, as the case may be.

This means that secretion is fully as important a part of the activity of a nerve cell as is its capacity to transmit nerve impulses, and it is therefore possible to interpret the chromaffin tissue as a further development of this secretory capacity, the cells concerned having lost the characteristic form of neurones and having come to specialize solely as secretory agents. This would clearly provide

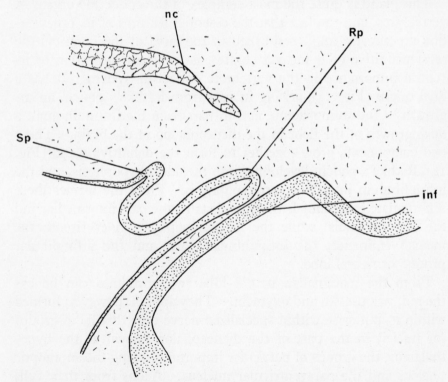

Fig. 13. Longitudinal section through the developing pituitary gland of a four-day duck embryo. *inf.*, floor of infundibulum; *nc.*, notochord; *Rp.*, Rathke's pouch; *Sp.*, Seessell's pouch (preoral gut).

another example of the possibility of a new function evolving by the intensification of an already existing function. It must not be assumed, however, that this interpretation is necessarily correct, for certain facts, arising out of studies of the chromaffin cells of lower vertebrates, are not easily reconciled with the view that these cells have evolved out of nervous tissue. It would take us too far afield to discuss this particular problem here, but the mere fact that endocrine and nervous tissue can produce an identical secretion is itself of considerable interest, for it suggests that the two co-ordinating systems may be more closely associated than is suggested by purely anatomical studies, and further evidence for this has been disclosed in recent studies of the organization of the pituitary gland.

This gland is quite the most complex of the endocrine organs of vertebrates, and the fact that the essential features of its organization are already fully established in the larva of the lamprey, the most primitive of living vertebrates, is sufficient indication of its central importance in the vertebrate endocrine system. It has a dual origin (Fig. 13), arising in part from Rathke's pouch, an ingrowth of the stomodaeum, and in part from the infundibulum, a downgrowth of the floor of the diencephalon of the brain. These two components grow together to form the definitive gland (Fig. 14), Rathke's pouch developing into the adenohypophysis, and the infundibulum into the neurohypophysis. From the former there differentiate in mammals the pars distalis, the pars intermedia, and the pars tuberalis, while the neurohypophysis gives rise to the median eminence, the infundibular stalk, and the infundibular process or neural lobe.

From the mammalian neural lobe two hormones can be extracted, vasopressin and oxytocin. They are not, however, formed within it, but arise within specialized nerve cells that lie in groups (or nuclei) in the part of the diencephalon known as the hypothalamus, the groups of particular importance being the supraoptic nucleus and the paraventricular nucleus. Axons from their cells extend into the neural lobe, and it is down certain of these that the hormones pass from the cell bodies in which they have been synthesized, the fibres having a characteristic varicose or beaded appearance because of the secretion within them (cf. Fig. 17). The hormones are then stored in the neural lobe, to be released

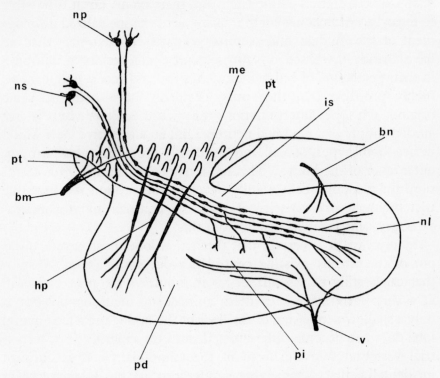

Fig. 14. The organization of the pituitary gland of mammals. Neurosecretory fibres from the supraoptic nucleus (*ns.*) and paraventricular nucleus (*np.*) run to the neural lobe (*nl.*); some have endings in the median eminence (*me.*) and pars intermedia (*pi.*). An arterial blood supply (*bm.*) gives vessels to capillary loops in the median eminence, from which the hypophyseal portal vessels (*hp.*) run to the pars distalis. The neural lobe receives a separate arterial blood supply (*bn.*). The venous blood is drained away at *v.*; *is.*, infundibular stalk; *pd.*, pars distalis; *pt.*, pars tuberalis. After figures by Harris, 1955, *The Neural Control of the Pituitary Gland* (London: Arnold).

into the blood stream as required, so that this region of the pituitary is not a secretory organ at all, but merely a storage and release centre. Such an organ is now known as a neurohaemal organ, because of the close functional relationship that it establishes between neural tissue and the vascular system.

The nerve cells that produce these hormones are referred to as neurosecretory cells. They are distinguishable by various characteristics, including the large size of their cell bodies and the presence of stainable secretion within them and their axons, but it is possible to regard them as being another example of the specialized development of the fundamental secretory capacity of neurones that we have already discussed. Neurosecretory cells resemble neurones in their possession of cell bodies, dendrites, and axons, and it seems highly probable that they must originally have had the same origin. On one interpretation the neurosecretory cell is regarded simply as a modified neurone, but an alternative view would derive both types of cell independently from the ectoderm, or outer layer of the body. This has a marked potentiality for secretion, for glandular cells readily develop from it, and it is possible that the secretory capacity of both the neurone and the neurosecretory cells takes its origin from this.

In any case, it is certain that the neural lobe must have evolved out of the already-existing central nervous system, and by steps that can readily be visualized, for in lampreys the process is still at a very early stage. In these animals the neurohypophysis is only a shallow depression of the floor of the brain, and a true neural lobe does not become differentiated until the emergence of terrestrial vertebrates in the form of the amphibians. It is curious, incidentally, that a somewhat similar process has taken place in fish, including both selachians and teleosts, at the hind end of the spinal cord. Neurosecretory cells are conspicuous in this region, and their nerve endings are associated with blood vessels in a swelling known as the urophysis (or urohypophysis) spinalis, which is undoubtedly another example of a neurohaemal organ. Its function is still obscure, although it is thought possibly to be involved in osmoregulation, but the formation of two such organs at opposite ends of the central nervous system is an illuminating example of similar structures arising independently by parallel evolution, not, as happens so often, in two different groups of animals, but in two different parts of the same body.

As regards the adenohypophysis of the pituitary gland, this has the typical histological structure of secretory tissue, so that its history has clearly been very different from that of the neurohypophysis. The pars intermedia of the adenohypophysis produces a secretion (melanocyte-stimulating hormone, or intermedin) that regulates colour change in the lower vertebrates (p. 113), and there is reason for believing that this region of the adenohypophysis is controlled by nerve fibres (perhaps neurosecretory ones) of the neurohypophysis. In the Amphibia these fibres seem to exert an inhibitory influence upon the pars intermedia, which develops into an unusually large size if it is separated from the neural lobe during larval development, and it may be that this control provides part of the explanation of the association of the adenohypophysis and the neurohypophysis, although we shall see that other factors are also involved in determining this relationship.

The pars distalis secretes six different hormones, and these we shall be considering later. It will be sufficient now to say that one is a growth hormone, and that five are referred to as tropic hormones (*trope*, turn). The activity of the tropic hormones, as their names suggests, is turned towards the regulation of the functioning of certain other endocrine glands. Corticotropin (ACTH) regulates the adrenocortical tissue, thyrotropin (thyroid-stimulating hormone, TSH) regulates the thyroid gland, while the remaining three, follicle-stimulating hormone (FSH), interstitial cell-stimulating hormone (ICSH, also known as luteinizing hormone, LH), and, at least in some species, prolactin, regulate the endocrine tissue of the gonads. These several tissues, then, the adrenocortical tissue, the thyroid, and the interstitial tissue of the gonads, may be regarded as the target organs of the tropic hormones of the pituitary. We may note in passing that the inter-relationship depends upon the principle known as negative feed-back, a term that has been taken over from the phraseology of engineering. The output of thyrotropin, for example, is itself regulated by the concentration of thyroid hormones circulating in the blood stream. If this concentration falls, the appropriate cells in the pars distalis respond by increasing their output of thyrotropin, and this stimulates the thyroid to increase its output of its own hormones. When the concentration of these in the blood stream has been restored to normal the pituitary cells will reduce their output of thyrotropin, and in this way all parts of the body are assured of a correctly balanced supply of thyroid secretion.

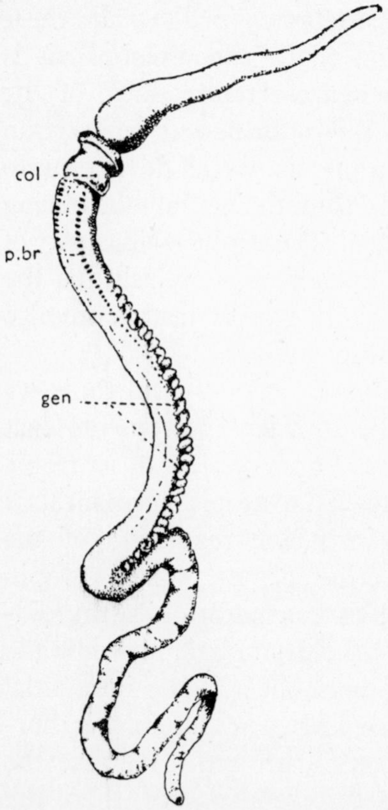

Since part of the function of the feed-back system is to adjust the output of the target glands to the changing demands imposed upon the animal by fluctuations of the internal and external environments, it is essential that the pituitary gland should itself be under the control of the central nervous system and thus in functional relationship with the receptor systems of the body. This control is not, however, effected by nerve fibres, but, as is now generally believed, by the passage of chemical transmitter substances through a specialized part of the blood system, the hypophyseal portal system (Fig. 14) that runs into the pars distalis from the median eminence in the floor of the diencephalon. The nature of these transmitter substances presents an interesting problem that we shall consider later, but the mere statement of the principle involved will sufficiently indicate why the association of the adenohypophysis with the floor of the brain is of such pre-eminent importance in vertebrate organization.

A study of the comparative anatomy of the pituitary gland shows that it has undergone considerable morphological and

Fig. 15. *Saccoglossus pusillus. col.* collar, in front of which extends the long proboscis; *p. br.*, branchial pores; *gen.*, genital pouches. From Dawydoff, 1948, in *Traité de Zoologie* (P.-P. Grassé, ed.), **11**, 369–532 (Paris: Masson).

histological specialization in the several classes of vertebrates, but this aspect of evolutionary history, fascinating and important though it is, lies outside the scope of our present discussion, for it tells us nothing at all of the possible origin of the adenohypophysis. As we have already remarked, the essential features of

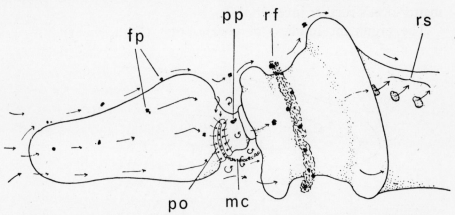

Fig. 16. Lateral view of the anterior end of *Protoglossus köhleri.* *fp.*, particles of sand and food which are collected in strands of mucus that are moved by ciliary action in the direction of the arrows; *mc.*, mucus strand from the preoral ciliary organ, *po.*; *pp.*, proboscis pore; *rf.*, particles which have not been ingested and which collect in bands of mucus around the collar; *rs.*, branchial pores, with outgoing current of water. From Burdon-Jones (1956), in *Handbuch der Zoologie* (Kükenthal and Krumbach, eds.), III, 2 (9), 57–78 (Berlin: de Gruyter).

pituitary organization are already clearly defined in the Cyclostomata, so that for light on its earlier evolutionary history we have to turn to the protochordates, without, however, expecting to find in these highly specialized animals a direct forerunner of the gland.

A fact that is highly suggestive from this point of view is a common tendency for a ciliated organ to form in the head region of these animals. The organs concerned are the preoral ciliary organ of *Saccoglossus* (Figs. 15 and 16) and related Hemichordata, the neural gland of Tunicata, and Hatschek's pit and the ciliated wheel organ of amphioxus (Fig. 17). The function of these several organs has still to be clarified, although there is a suggestion that the hemichordate one may be sensory, and that in the Tunicata the neural gland may play some part in the co-ordination of reproductive activity by virtue of its sensitivity to the sex products of other individuals. It is thought that these may stimulate the gland, and that this in its turn could then evoke in some way the release of germ cells from its own body. The present evidence does not justify pressing this argument very far, and the whole matter needs further investigation.

The argument implies, of course, that the adenohypophysis

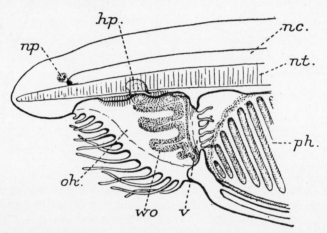

Fig. 17. Left side view of the head of a young amphioxus. The left body wall, oral hood, and wall of the pharynx have been cut away. *hp.*, Hatschek's pit; *nc.*, nerve cord; *np.*, Kölliker's pit; *nt.*, notochord; *ph.*, pharynx; *oh.*, oral hood; *wo.*, wheel organ; *v.*, velum. From Goodrich, 1917, *Quart. J. micr. Sci.*, **62**, 539–553.

might have evolved as a further specialization of an already existing secretory structure, and there is one piece of evidence that supports this view. Hatschek's pit and the wheel organ arise from the preoral pit of the larval amphioxus, and this pit has an opening into the most anterior of the segmental coelomic pouches. A precisely similar opening, or a closed vestige of it, appears also during the development of Rathke's pouch in certain higher vertebrates (it has been recorded both in a fish and in a bird), and it is difficult to account for such an extraordinary similarity except on the assumption that this pouch must be homologous with Hatschek's pit and the wheel organ. These structures contain secretory cells, so that there does seem to be a case for deriving the adeno-hypophysis from a cephalic glandular organ, although we can do little more than guess what circumstances might have determined the evolution of such an organ into the adenohypophysis as we see it today.

In view of what has been said above regarding the possible function of the neural gland of tunicates, however, it is worth noting that the very real importance of chemical communication between individuals of a species has been increasingly realized in recent years, one of the most closely studied examples of this being the 'queen substance' of bee colonies. This is a substance secreted by the queen and distributed throughout the colony by the workers, its physiological effect being to inhibit the latter from making queen cells and rearing queens, while it also prevents the development in them of fertile ovaries. In the absence of a queen no such substance will, of course, be available; in such circumstances the workers will, therefore, begin to rear new queens, and thus provision is made for the continued fertility of the colony. There is clearly a close analogy between such substances and hormones, the fundamental difference lying in the external distribution of the former. They are now usually referred to as ecto-hormones (or pheromones), and it is interesting to speculate on the possibility of some evolutionary relationship between this type of mechanism and the internal mode of operation of the classical hormones, although we have as yet no positive evidence of such a relationship. All that we can say is that a cephalic sensory organ, sensitive to the environment or to the products of other individuals, and capable of releasing chemical signals, might have become sensitive to the products of its own body, and this gives us some basis for visualizing a possible mode of origin of the far-reaching internal regulatory power that the pars distalis now possesses.

The Endocrine Systems of Invertebrates

In our later discussion of molecular structure we shall be concerned almost exclusively with vertebrate hormones, for too little is

known of the invertebrate ones to justify much generalization in
this field. The structural organization of the endocrine systems
of invertebrates has, however, been very thoroughly investigated
in recent years, and the result has been to disclose remarkable
parallelisms between the organization and modes of functioning of
these systems in different groups of the animal kingdom.

This phenomenon of the evolution of similar adaptations from
different origins is often referred to as convergence, and it provides examples of analogy, this term being applied to resemblances
between structures that have been evolved independently in unrelated groups of animals and that owe their similarities to the
common functions that they subserve. We customarily contrast
analogy with homology, the classical post-Darwinian tradition
being to term structures homologous when they are considered to
have had their origin in a structure present in some remote common ancestor of the groups concerned.

The considerations involved here, however, are subtle ones. We
have seen in our reference to the B vitamins that important features
of metabolic pathways, established at a very early stage of evolution,
may subsequently be incorporated into quite diverse groups of
organisms, and we have noted, too, how patterns of metabolism
and differentiation may be direct expressions of gene action. This
suggests that similarities of organization may sometimes owe their
existence not to their derivation from structures already present in
a common ancestor, but to the inheritance by the groups concerned
of some common genetic potentiality or biochemical capacity.
Given similar adaptational requirements, therefore, it may well
happen in these circumstances that remarkably similar features
will appear independently in quite different groups of animals.
Structures arising in this way are often described as homoplastic, or
are said to illustrate latent homology, and it seems likely that this
type of relationship is involved in the parallelisms that are now being
disclosed in the neurosecretory systems of certain groups of animals.

Neurosecretory cells are widely distributed through the invertebrates, and are often so abundant as to suggest that the central
nervous system must be regarded as a major endocrine system.

Why this should be so is not clear, although it must reflect in some way or other the evolutionary history of these cells. We have already noted the suggestion that nerve cells and neurosecretory cells may owe their secretory properties to their derivation from the ectoderm. On this view it could be argued that the prevalence of neurosecretory cells in the nervous systems of the lower invertebrates is a consequence of the primitive nature of these systems themselves, and of the close relationships that they often still maintain with surface epithelia. In higher forms they would tend to become more localized and specialized in their relationships as the nervous system underwent further evolution.

However this may be, it is certainly a fact that cells with the appearance of neurosecretory cells are conspicuous in the cerebral ganglia of annelid worms, for instance, and their axons have been traced in the polychaete *Nephtys* (*Nephthys*) to the vascular membrane surrounding the ganglia, which seems to form a primitive type of neurohaemal organ. These cells seem to be deeply implicated in the regulation of the growth and reproduction of polychaetes. For example, the capacity to regenerate the hind end of the body is seriously impaired in *Nephtys* if the cerebral ganglia are removed. Particularly striking, however, is their influence upon the reproductive cycle of nereid worms, many of which become modified into a heteronereid phase when they are sexually mature. In this phase the hinder end of the body, called the epitoke, contains the ripe germ cells, and is structurally modified in various ways, as, for example, in the form of its parapodia, while there are also modifications at the anterior end, such as the enlargement of the eyes. There is now good evidence that in immature worms the neurosecretory cells of the cerebral ganglia are exerting an inhibitory influence upon sexual maturation, for if these ganglia are removed from an immature specimen this will rapidly advance to sexual maturity. Moreover, implantation of the ganglia into worms that, as a result of decerebration, would otherwise become sexually mature, will delay or inhibit the establishment of that condition.

Neurosecretory cells are present, too, in the cerebral ganglia of

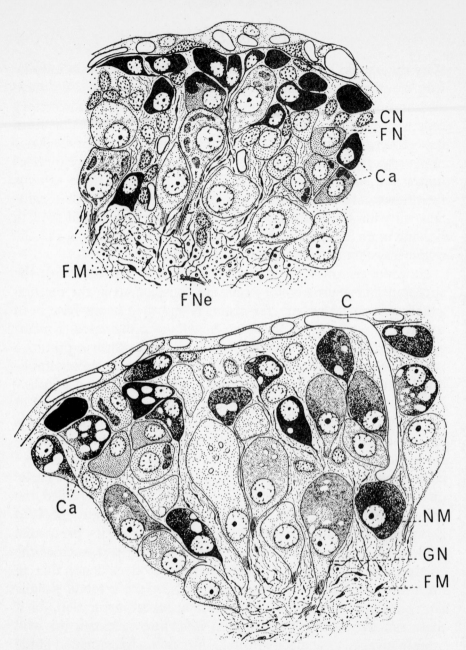

Fig. 18. *Above*, section through the posterior part of the supraoesophageal gang-lion of a 48-mm. earthworm, *Eisenia foetida*. *Below*, a similar section from a mature specimen that had laid forty-seven cocoons, and in which the neuro-secretory cells are much vacuolated. *C.*, capillaries; *Ca.*, neurosecretory cells; *CN.*, neuroglia cells; *FM.*, neurosecretory fibres, their contained secretion giving them a moniliform appearance; *FN.*, neuroglia fibres; *FNe.*, nerve fibres; *GN.*, large neurone; *NM.*, medium neurone. From Herlant-Meewis, 1956, *Ann. Sci. Nat. Zool. 11 sér., 18*, 185–198.

earthworms (Fig. 18), where also they are believed to influence the reproductive cycle, not, however, by inhibition, as in nereids, but by promoting the development of secondary sexual characters such as the clitellum.   This is of particular interest in showing that the evolution of similar endocrine systems, even in groups as closely related as polychaetes and oligochaetes, may yet be accompanied by important divergences in structure or in mode of functioning, divergences that are doubtless related in some way to the adaptational requirements of the groups concerned.

The same point is illustrated in the arthropods, particularly if we compare the insects and crustaceans with each other and with the vertebrates.   The two former groups are, of course, closely related, but they have had a long period of independent evolution, their divergence having presumably taken place at least 500 million years ago, for crustaceans were already well differentiated in the Cambrian period.   While, therefore, we may expect them to show some measure of homology, either latent or overt, there is clearly much scope for the development of analogous features by convergence, and this needs to be borne in mind when comparing their endocrine systems.

As for the vertebrates, these animals are quite remote from the arthropods, so that we necessarily look for analogy rather than for homology in comparing them with the latter.   Nevertheless, both vertebrates and arthropods make use of neurosecretory cells, so that we shall expect to find that the properties of these, and their inevitable demand for neurohaemal release centres, will impose common features of organization and will thereby lead to the independent evolution of systems that may come to bear very close resemblances to each other.   It would be straining the term homology too much to apply it to such situations, yet it is clear that these resemblances, traceable as they are to roots lying deep in the organization of metazoan animals, are something more than the wholly unrelated analogies of classical morphology.   It is in such respects that an increased understanding of the principles of animal structure and function demand an increasing flexibility in our analysis of them.

Insects and crustaceans, like the vertebrates, have very well-developed neurosecretory systems, too complex both in organization and in functioning to be mentioned here in more than brief outline. Neurosecretory cells are found in the brain of insects in a dorso-medial region called the pars intercerebralis, and discharge their secretion down axons into a neurohaemal organ, the corpus cardiacum (Fig. 18). Included in this secretion is a hormone called the prothoracotropic hormone, the function of which is to stimulate the prothoracic gland to discharge its growth and moulting hormone. This initiates the sequence of growth and moulting that is a familiar feature of arthropods, and that is imposed upon them by their possession of a rigid skeleton. The parallel with vertebrates is here a close one, as far as organization is concerned, for the relation between the brain and corpus cardiacum is precisely the same as that between the hypothalamic nuclei and the neural lobe.

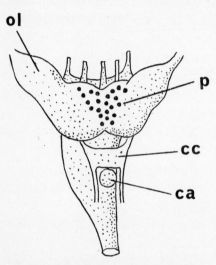

Fig. 19. Some features of the endocrine system of a larval insect, *Rhodnius. ca.*, corpus allatum; *cc.*, corpus cardiacum; *ol.*, optic lobe; *p.*, protocerebrum. Neurosecretory cells lie centrally in the pars intercerebralis, and their position is indicated approximately by the coarse stippling. After Wigglesworth, 1940, *J. exp. Biol.*, **17**, 201–222.

Moreover, there is in insects another gland, the corpus allatum (Fig. 19), that is closely associated with the corpus cardiacum, much as the adenohypophysis is with the neural lobe, and which is involved in much the same functional relationship, for it is regulated by the brain, probably by nerve fibres that reach it through the corpus cardiacum. Nevertheless, these resemblances have been independently developed in unrelated groups, and we are reminded of this by the mode of action of the corpus allatum, which differs in an interesting way from that of the adenohypophysis. The former secretes a hormone called the juvenile hormone, the presence of which during larval life prevents the establishment of adult characters at the moult, and to this function there is no exact parallel in the vertebrates, or, indeed, in any other group of animals so far studied.

This same pattern of interlocking resemblances and differences is found when we compare the crustacean endocrine system with that of the vertebrates. Neurosecretory cells are prominent in

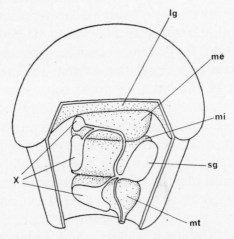

Fig. 20. Dorsal dissection of the left eye stalk of the prawn, *Pandalus borealis*, simplified. The medulla terminalis (*mt.*) is a brain centre, while the medulla interna (*mi.*), medulla externa (*me.*) and lamina ganglionaris (*lg.*) are optic centres. Neurosecretory cells in the three X organs (X) give off tracts of fibres that run to a neurohaemal organ, the sinus gland (*sg.*). Redrawn from Carlisle, 1959, *J. mar. biol. Ass. U.K.*, **38**, 381–394.

various parts of the central nervous system of the higher crustaceans, certain groups in the region of the brain forming the so-called X organs (Fig. 20), which may be compared with the pars intercerebralis of insects. The corresponding neurohaemal organs for this cerebral system are the sinus gland, usually to be found in the eye stalk, alongside a blood sinus, and the post-commissure organ, associated with the circumoesophageal connectives and the post-oesophageal commissure. These clearly correspond closely with the corpus cardiacum of insects as far as their relationships with the brain are concerned, although their positions in the body are markedly different.

The hormones produced in the neurosecretory centres of crustaceans are probably many and diverse, but some are certainly concerned with the regulation of colour change.   Here we find a good example of the differences between the modes of functioning of the endocrine systems of invertebrates and vertebrates, for, as we have seen, colour change in the latter is regulated by an adenohypophyseal hormone and not by a neurosecretory product, although the release of that hormone is probably under neurosecretory control. On the other hand, the stick insect *Carausius* (*Dixippus*), one of the very few insects to show colour change comparable to that of crustaceans, possesses a regulating system sufficiently similar in principle to that of the latter group to suggest that we are here dealing with a substantial element of homology.   Not only is the colour change of *Carausius* regulated, at least in part, by a neurosecretory product of the central nervous system, but the similarity may lie even deeper than this, for there is some evidence of a measure of chemical identity of the hormones of the two groups, a point that we shall refer to again at a later stage (p. 119).   For the moment it will be evident that this comparison of the regulation of colour change in crustaceans, insects, and vertebrates shows that the first two of these groups resemble each other much more closely than either of them resemble the vertebrates, a conclusion that is in full accord with our earlier discussion of the implications of the evolutionary relationships of these animals.

No less striking is the fact that moulting in crustaceans is regulated through the sinus gland, which functions in this instance like the corpus cardiacum of insects, releasing a tropic hormone which then controls the activity of an endocrine gland called the Y organ. There seems here to be a close parallel between this organ and the prothoracic gland of insects; indeed, the two are possibly homologous, although there is an important difference in their mode of functioning which doubtless reflects the long period of independent evolution of the two groups.   The growth and moulting hormone of the prothoracic gland activates the moulting process, whereas the moulting hormone of the Y organ inhibits it, so that the tropic hormone of insects stimulates the release of an activator, whereas that of crustaceans inhibits the release of an inhibitor. The result is essentially the same, but the mechanism different, and there could be no better illustration of the care with which interpretations of evolutionary relationships have to be approached. The most successful of detective-story writers would be likely to be out-matched by the skill with which nature confuses the trail at the least expected moment!

It should be remembered that this note of excitement is inherent in the process of natural selection. This is not a creative agent in the sense of being able to determine the type of mutation that will emerge in a particular group at a particular time. What it does do is to exert a directive influence by selecting advantageous muta-tions from among the many presented to it. Operating in this way over vast periods of time, and with a wide range of variation at its disposal, it generates the very high degree of improbability that we noted at the beginning of this discussion, an improbability shown in the perfection of adaptation achieved from unpromising beginnings, and in the startling convergences that we have just been outlining.

With these reflections we have perhaps seen enough, brief though the view has been, to suggest the ready possibility of interpreting endocrine systems as products of long evolutionary processes, often derivable with reasonable plausibility from pre-existing fea-tures of organization without the necessity for postulating sudden and drastic change. Nevertheless, it will have become evident that analysis at the morphological level leaves many questions un-answered, and that we need to extend our understanding by probing deeper into the nature and history of the hormones themselves, and of the metabolic pathways through which they originate. It will now be our purpose, therefore, to enquire whether the principles of evolutionary theory operate as clearly at the molecular level as they seem to do at the morphological one.

2 *The Steroid Hormones*

We do the thing pleasantly and in a great variety of styles, and are generally considered to make it as agreeable as possible to the feelings of the survivors. But don't obtrude it, don't obtrude it. Easy, easy!
Charles Dickens: *Martin Chuzzlewit*

Sterols and the Steroid Nucleus

IT has long been known that the response of fats (lipids) to treatment with alkali makes it possible to distinguish them into two groups. Members of one of these groups can be converted to water-soluble substances by alkaline hydrolysis, a process called saponification, whereas those of the other group resist such treatment and are referred to as non-saponifiable lipids.

Included in the latter group are the substances known as sterols. These are secondary alcohols with molecules containing 27 to 29 carbon atoms, and they exist as crystalline solids (*stereos*, solid) with melting points ranging from about 100° to 200° C. Probably the best known of all sterols is cholesterol, a substance to which we have already referred, and which is the main constituent of the gall-stones that are so readily deposited in the bile-ducts of human beings (*chole*, bile). Its molecular formula is $C_{27}H_{45}OH$, so that it is known as a C_{27} sterol, and it has the molecular structure illustrated conventionally in Fig. 21. It will be observed that the nucleus of this structure is a four-membered ring, and this is called the cyclopentenoperhydrophenanthrene system. All substances containing this nucleus in their molecules are referred to as steroids, a term that includes not only the sterols themselves but also many other biologically important substances, among which are a number of vertebrate hormones.

Steroids are remarkably diverse in their biological properties, and

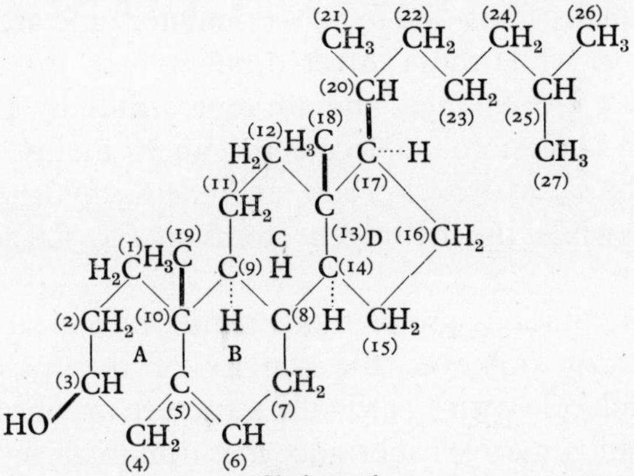

Fig. 21. Conventional diagram of the structure of the cholesterol molecule.

this diversity, in itself a fact of the greatest evolutionary importance, depends upon a corresponding diversity in the details of their molecular structure, to which, therefore, we must pay some attention. As may be seen from Fig. 21, the steroid nucleus can carry substituent groups attached at points that are identified by a conventional system of numbering of the carbon atoms. In the cholesterol molecule there are methyl groups attached at C_{10} (i.e. at the carbon atom bearing the number 10) and C_{13}, and a hydroxyl group at C_3, while the second ring (ring B) is unsaturated, with a double bond at the C_5–C_6 position. Further, C_{17} bears a complex side chain with 8 carbon atoms.

We shall see many examples of the ways in which alterations in the substituent groups or in the side chain bring about changes in the biological activity of steroid molecules, but in considering such alterations it is necessary to remember that these molecules are three-dimensional structures, and that their conventional two-dimensional representations are misleadingly simple in appearance. For our present purpose it will be sufficient to say that the nucleus may be regarded as being relatively flat, with its substituent groups lying either in the same plane as itself, in which case their bonds are described as equatorial, or vertical to it, in which case they are described as axial. Axial bonds directed upwards (i.e. above the plane of the nucleus) are said to be β-orientated, and are represented by a thick line, while those directed downwards (below the plane of the ring) are α-orientated, and are represented by a broken line. Thus, in the cholesterol molecule the angle methyl groups, the side chain, the C_3 hydroxyl group, and the C_8 hydrogen atom are β-orientated, while the hydrogen atoms at C_9, C_{14}, and C_{17} are α-orientated.

These configurations are of fundamental biological importance, for they directly influence the activity of the molecules. For example, a molecule with a particular structure may be active, while its epimer (which means a substance identical in all respects except that one group, α- or β-orientated, is replaced by one with the opposite orientation) may be inactive (p. 53). Perhaps such alterations vary the ease with which a steroid molecule can interact with other molecules or can enter into functional relationship with, for example, the surface membranes of particular types of cell.

As regards the sterols themselves, cholesterol is the only one of major importance in the vertebrates, and, indeed, its presence is a clearly defined biochemical characteristic of the group. It is particularly abundant in the nervous system, as well as in gall-stones, but it appears to be a constituent of all the tissues, as much as 140 g being present in a man weighing about 70 kg. Part of its function is probably to contribute to the structure of the cell membranes that have been shown by the electron microscope to be an important feature of the architecture of the cell, but it is also an active metabolite, and is a stage in the synthesis of other important products, including some, and perhaps all, of the steroid hormones that we are to discuss.

In other groups of animals, as well as in plants, sterols seem to be no less essential constituents of the tissues, but they vary a great deal in their structure. Cholesterol is often present in invertebrates and in the Protozoa, but it is accompanied by many other related compounds, some of which may be restricted to particular groups. For example, the sterols of the barnacle *Balanus glandula* include cholesterol to the extent of 60%, together with 34% of its derivative, 24-dehydrocholesterol (Fig. 22), while from the sponge

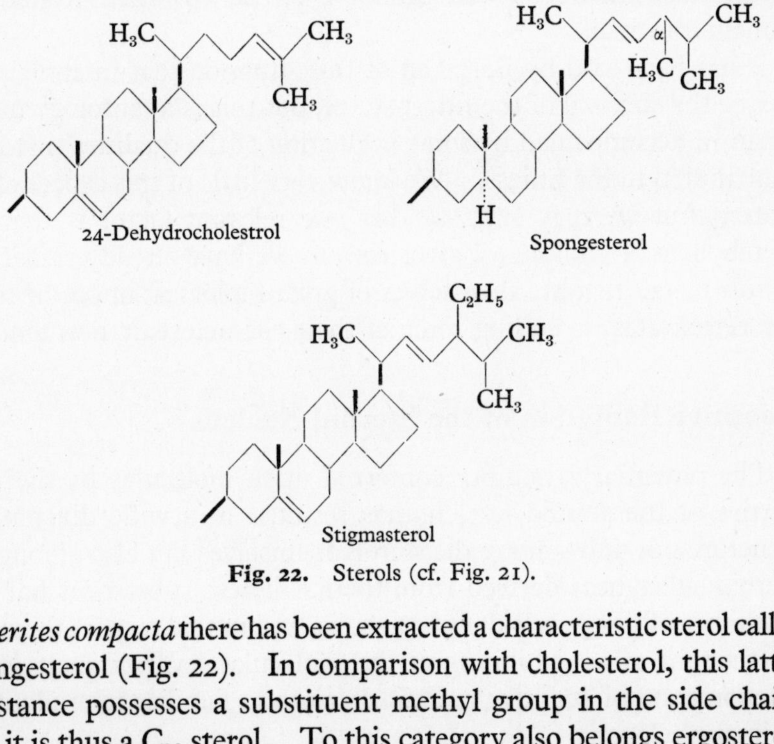

24-Dehydrocholestrol

Spongesterol

Stigmasterol

Fig. 22.   Sterols (cf. Fig. 21).

Suberites compacta there has been extracted a characteristic sterol called spongesterol (Fig. 22). In comparison with cholesterol, this latter substance possesses a substituent methyl group in the side chain, and it is thus a C_{28} sterol. To this category also belongs ergosterol, which is found in yeast and in the mould *Neurospora*. This is a sterol of particular interest because, as we have seen, it gives rise to vitamin D_2 when it is irradiated with ultraviolet light. Finally, C_{29} sterols are particularly characteristic of the higher plants, stigmasterol (Fig. 22), obtained from soya-bean oil, being a typical representative.

It is thus clear that there has been, so to speak, a good deal of experimentation with sterol structure in the course of evolution.

There is evidence, too, that lower organisms, such as the sponges, synthesize a greater diversity of these substances than do the higher ones, and we must certainly suppose that the natural selection of cholesterol as the characteristic sterol of vertebrates was made from out of a wide range of possibilities. Moreover, this selection must have been achieved at an early stage in the evolution of the group, for the C_{28} and C_{29} sterols cannot be metabolized at all by its present-day members, and cannot even be absorbed from their alimentary canal.

It has been said by Bergman of this situation that in cholesterol we see the survival of the fittest sterol, but this is a tautology unless it can be accompanied by some evaluation of the qualities that have contributed to the fitness. We know very little of this aspect of the matter, but we may suppose that one relevant factor is that the metabolism of cholesterol gives rise, as we have already remarked, to substances that are themselves of great biological importance for the vertebrates, including some of their characteristic hormones.

Adaptive Radiation of the Steroid Nucleus

The potential variability conferred upon molecules by the properties of the steroid nucleus has resulted in a wide diversity of structure not only among the sterols themselves but also among the steroid substances derived from them. These substances fall into a number of fairly well-defined groups, and in this respect they may be thought of as exhibiting at the molecular level of analysis the phenomenon of adaptive radiation that is so familiar to students of animal phylogeny.

For example, many plants contain steroids that are combined with carbohydrate to form glycosides, these including the surface-active agents (detergents) known as neutral saponins which produce foam in water. Others, the cardiotonic glycosides, have a stimulating action on the heart, and are the source of the important medical agent known as digitalin obtained from foxgloves, while in the form of native arrow poisons they will arrest the heart beat as a result of over-stimulation. Related to these cardiotonic substances are other steroids that are found in free or conjugated form in the venom that is secreted by the parotid glands of toads, an example being bufotalin, which carries an acetyl group at C_{16}.

Particularly instructive steroids from our present point of view are the bile salts of vertebrates, substances that make an important contribution to the course of digestion by their emulsification of fats and by the activation of the pancreatic lipase that hydrolyses the latter. The common bile acids of mammals, from which these salts are derived, are C_{24} steroids, and they are known to be formed by the metabolism of cholesterol, this giving rise in man to several bile acids of which cholic acid is an example. Here again there is much variation between species, and higher vertebrates may have characteristic C_{24} bile acids, such as the hyocholic acid of the pig and the pythocholic acid of the python.

More striking than this diversification of the C_{24} compounds, however, is the fact that lower vertebrates have bile steroids that differ from those of higher forms in the possession of more carbon atoms. In the bile of elasmobranchs, for example, there is a sulphate ester of a steroid substance called scymnol (after the shark *Scymnus borealis* from which it was first prepared); this is a C_{27} steroid with the formula $C_{27}H_{46}O_5$, and it apparently takes the place of the more familiar bile salts of mammals. Similarly, the carp, *Cyprinus carpio*, has cyprinol, $C_{27}H_{43}(OH)_5$, and the common frog, *Rana temporaria*, ranol, $C_{27-28}H_{43-45}(OH)_5$, while the crocodile has trihydroxycoprostanic acid, $C_{27}H_{46}O_5$, which is also present in the frog.

These C_{27} and C_{28} compounds are probably derived, like the C_{24} ones, from cholesterol, but it is suggested that the degradation of the side chain of its molecule is arrested, so to speak, at an early stage. On this view the resulting compounds may be regarded as primitive, just as characters like a persistent notochord are regarded as primitive at the morphological level of analysis. We may suppose, therefore, that the capacity for achieving full oxidation of the side chain of cholesterol, with the production of the typical C_{24} bile acids of mammals, is a specialized feature of the more advanced vertebrates.

These considerations, brief though they have been, will serve to illustrate the remarkable evolutionary potentialities of the steroid nucleus. We cannot doubt that natural selection has been able to act upon its variant forms, resulting in the existence today of primitive and specialized levels of differentiation, and in the accumulation of specific or group differences between related forms. In such ways molecular evolution seems to follow paths closely comparable with those familiar to students of comparative anatomy. We have, therefore, some justification for our hope that studies of the molecular structure of hormones may be no less helpful than studies of anatomical structure in providing illustrations of evolution in action, and we may expect such studies to provide further clarification of the evolutionary history of endocrine systems.

The Steroid Hormones of Vertebrates

The steroid hormones of vertebrates are formed in one or other of three regions, the placenta, the gonads, and the adrenocortical tissue, and we have seen that these are linked by a close developmental relationship with the coelomic epithelium. The hormones themselves have characteristic differences in their molecular structure (Fig. 23), and these can be correlated with differences in their biological activities, a fact that has facilitated the synthesis of substances identical with, or related to, the naturally occurring products. Both natural products and synthetic ones, however, can be broadly classified on structural and functional criteria into three groups, the oestrogens, the androgens, and the corticosteroids, the natural members of each group being primarily secreted by one particular tissue. This latter distinction is not absolute, however, and we shall see that steroid hormones of one group may be present in a tissue that is primarily concerned with the secretion of another group.

The most potent of the oestrogens is oestradiol-17β (commonly referred to simply as oestradiol), which is secreted by the mammalian ovary, and, in certain species, by the placenta; it may be regarded as the chief sex hormone of the female mammal, being

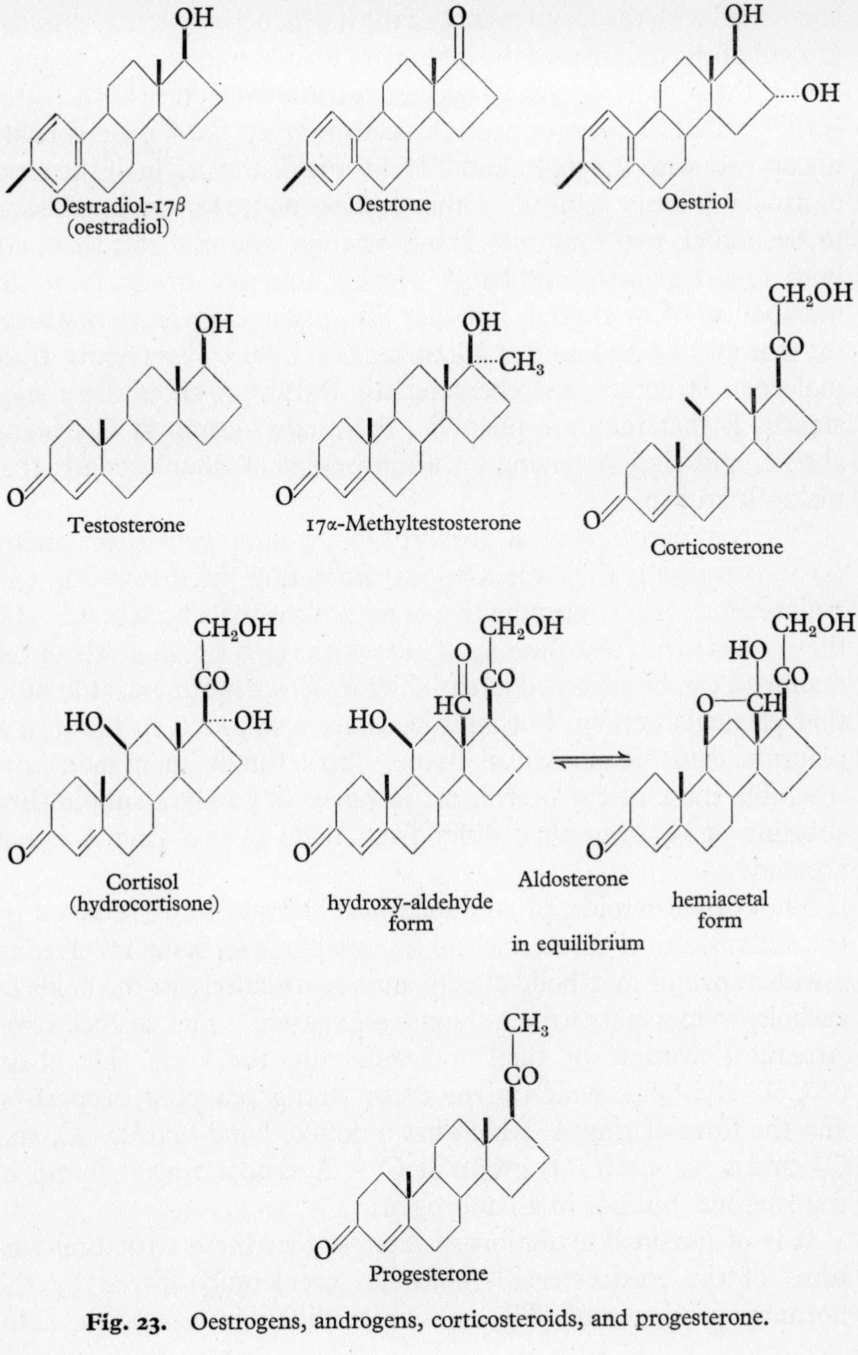

Fig. 23. Oestrogens, androgens, corticosteroids, and progesterone.

concerned with the maintenance of the reproductive organs, with the growth of the ductules of the mammary glands, and with the regulation of the sexual or oestrous cycle. A common feature of the latter is the periodical onset of heat, or oestrus, when the female is ready to copulate with the male, and it is this that is the origin of the term oestrogen (*oistros*, gadfly). Other oestrogens are known in addition to oestradiol, two examples being oestrone and oestriol; these are both found in urine, probably because they are products of the metabolism of oestradiol, but they also occur elsewhere, oestrone, for example, being found in adrenocortical tissue. As regards their molecular structure, the characteristic feature of all of these substances is that they are phenolic, the methyl group at C_{10} being absent, and ring A having an arrangement of double bonds that makes it aromatic.

The common biological property of the androgens (*aner*, male; *genos*, descent) is their capacity for promoting the maturation and maintenance of the reproductive organs of the male vertebrate. Of these substances, testosterone, which is secreted by the testis of the mammal, can be regarded as the chief male sex hormone, at least in that particular group, but androgens are also found in the ovary, placenta, and adrenocortical tissue. Structurally their molecules resemble those of the oestrogens in possessing only a simple substitution at C_{17}, but they differ from them in that ring A is not aromatic.

The corticosteroids, or adrenocortical hormones, are secreted by the adrenocortical tissue, and are essential for life, being involved in a wide range of metabolic effects, more particularly in the fields of carbohydrate metabolism and ionic regulation. The characteristic structural features of their molecules are the ketol side chain ($-CO-CH_2OH$), which gives them strong reducing properties, and the form of ring A, which has a double bond between C_4 and C_5, and a ketone ($C:O$) group at C_3. A similar ring is found in testosterone, but not in all androgens.

It is of no small evolutionary interest that these structural features of the corticosteroid molecules are largely shared by the hormone progesterone (Fig. 23), which differs in lacking the ketol group in the side chain. Its position in this respect is somewhat anomalous, for progesterone is a mammalian sex hormone that differs profoundly from the adrenocortical hormones in its physiological role. It is characteristic of the female placental mammals that when the egg is shed from the Graafian follicle the latter is transformed into an endocrine gland, the corpus luteum, which secretes progesterone. One function of this hormone is to promote proliferation of the uterine lining, and thereby to prepare it for the reception of the fertilized egg; further, it is responsible for the maintenance of pregnancy (being, in fact, secreted also by the placenta in some species), while it prepares for the suckling of the young by promoting proliferation of the alveoli of the mammary glands. These functions, being peculiar to mammals, must have been established late in vertebrate evolution, and we shall consider later the way in which the appropriate hormonal control may have evolved.

It would be possible to pursue the molecular analysis of the steroid hormones much further, for within each group it can be shown that modifications of the basic molecular structure markedly influence biological activity. Testosterone, for example, is the most active of the naturally occurring androgens, and possesses at C_{17} a hydroxyl group in the β position, but its synthetic epimer *epi*testosterone, which differs from it only in having this group in the α position, is much less active. 17α-methyltestosterone (Fig. 23) will serve for another example. This is an androgen that carries an additional group at C_{17} in the α position, and it has a high potency, higher even than that of testosterone when taken by mouth. 17β-methyltestosterone, however, which differs only in the reversed orientation of the methyl group, is quite inactive.

There are, then, remarkable possibilities of variation within the basic molecular structure of the steroid hormones, and it is not surprising to find that many steroid substances have been extracted from the glands concerned, more particularly from the adrenocortical tissue. It is to be remembered, however, that not all of these are necessarily hormones. Some may arise as artifacts of the extraction procedures, while even when certain of them are known to be present within the gland it by no means follows that they are released into the circulation, for they may be no more than steps in the biosynthesis of the actual hormones themselves.

This position can best be understood by considering in outline some of the metabolic pathways that are believed to be involved in the production of the steroid hormones (Fig. 24). We have already

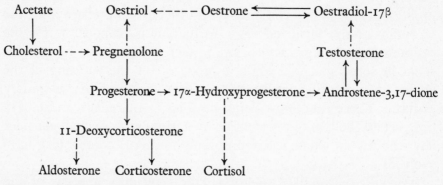

Fig. 24. Metabolic pathways that are thought to be involved in the biosynthesis of steroid hormones. Broken lines indicate that more than one step is involved. It is possible that cholesterol is not always an obligatory precursor, but that similar compounds can substitute for it. Simplified from Samuels, 1960, in *Metabolic Pathways* (B. M. Greenberg ed.), Vol. 1, (New York: Academic Press).

mentioned in this connexion the importance of cholesterol, the synthesis of which, probably from acetate, is thought to be the first stage in the production of the corticosteroids and possibly of all the steroid hormones, although the place of cholesterol may sometimes be taken by compounds closely related to it. Subsequent stages then involve successive structural changes in the molecule, changes that are believed to be catalysed by appropriate enzymes.

In this way cholesterol is thought to be transformed into progesterone, through the intermediary pregnenolone, by partial degradation of its side chain; from progesterone are then derived the characteristic hormones of the adrenocortical tissue, these being formed by hydroxylation at C_{21}, and also, according to the particular hormone concerned, at C_{11} and C_{17}. Acetate and cholesterol are also precursors of the androgens, so that the production of these hormones is linked with the metabolic pathways of the corticosteroids. This is probably true also of the oestrogens, which are thought possibly to be derived from progesterone through testosterone, by the hydroxylation of the angle methyl group at C_{19}, and by modification of ring A to the aromatic form.

This production of steroid hormones by stepwise synthesis, and the interlocking of the relevant metabolic pathways, goes some way to explain why as many as seventy different steroids have been isolated from adrenocortical extracts. It also makes it easier to understand why active substances can be obtained from what are, so to speak, the wrong sources. Oestrone, for example, has been obtained from the urine of stallions, and oestradiol from the testis of various vertebrates. Moreover, as many as eight androgenic steroids, including testosterone, have been identified in adrenocortical extracts. It would appear, in fact, that not only can compounds with one type of activity be converted into those of another type, as shown in Fig. 24, but that the glandular tissues themselves are by no means restricted to only one path of biosynthesis. It has, indeed, been suggested that any tissue capable of synthesizing steroid hormones is qualitatively much the same in its properties as any other such tissue. This would mean that the specialized properties of the endocrine cells concerned are manifested in purely quantitative differences in the main products that they secrete, differences that might well depend on nothing more complex than the relative strengths of the enzymes that catalyse the structural alterations in the molecules.

Such a view may be going rather further than the facts justify, but the steroid-secreting tissues certainly seem to retain capacities that exceed their obvious requirements, and this is in itself a situation needing explanation. We are at present in no position to provide this, but certain considerations are worth bearing in mind. It is possible that the production of, so to say, unnecessary types of molecule may simply mean that they are inevitable by-products of the successive steps that are involved in steroid synthesis. In genetic terms, we might say that they are pleiotropic effects of genes that have been selected primarily for the production of certain biologically important molecules. On the other hand, it may

c

perfectly well be that these molecules have functions that have not yet been detected; for example, their production may serve to vary or modulate the effects of the primary hormones, and so make possible a more refined control of the biological processes that they are regulating. We simply do not understand these matters at this stage, nor is this surprising when it is borne in mind that the structure of the steroid molecule was established only some twenty-five years ago.

What we can safely say, however, is that the orderly production of steroid hormones within the vertebrate must be thought of as the result of the favouring by natural selection of certain paths of bio-synthesis out of an originally much wider range of possibilities. Against this background, then, we can proceed to look a little more closely at some problems of their evolutionary history, and here two particular questions suggest themselves. First, are these very characteristic vertebrate hormones to be regarded as true evolutionary novelties, or are they foreshadowed in other organisms than the vertebrates? Second, to what extent, if any, have these molecules, once established in the group, undergone further evolution in relation to the greatly changing adaptational needs which must have arisen during the course of vertebrate history?

Evolution and the Sex Steroids

As regards the first of the above questions, we have already noted the existence, throughout the living world, of a wide diversity of sterol metabolism, and it would seem reasonable to infer from this that some at least of the biologically active steroids of vertebrates might well have been in existence in advance of the vertebrates themselves. Unfortunately, our information in this field is very limited, but it is none the less sufficient to indicate some justification for this inference, if only with respect to the oestrogens.

Thus, oestrogenic activity has been detected in plant material, oestrone having been extracted from palm kernels, and oestriol from the female catkins of the willow. Whether these substances are of any functional importance in the plants concerned is quite unknown, but it may well be, of course, that they are chance by-products of sterol metabolism. It is perhaps significant in this connexion that oestriol, formed from oestradiol by a hydroxylase, is the least active of the three main oestrogens of mammals, and is almost certainly a degradation product, obtainable from urine and placental tissue, but not from ovaries. Moreover, oestradiol, the most active oestrogen in mammals, and the one that is secreted by the ovaries, has not yet been identified in plants.

Oestrogenic activity has also been detected in certain invertebrate animals, but it must be emphasized that this is not in itself adequate evidence for the presence in them of steroid molecules. The difficulty here is that although the biological activity of a molecule can

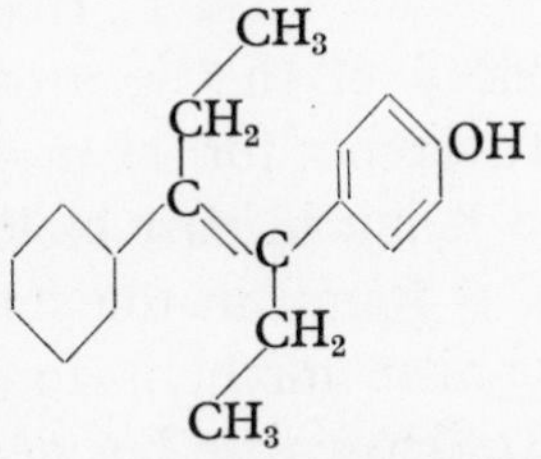

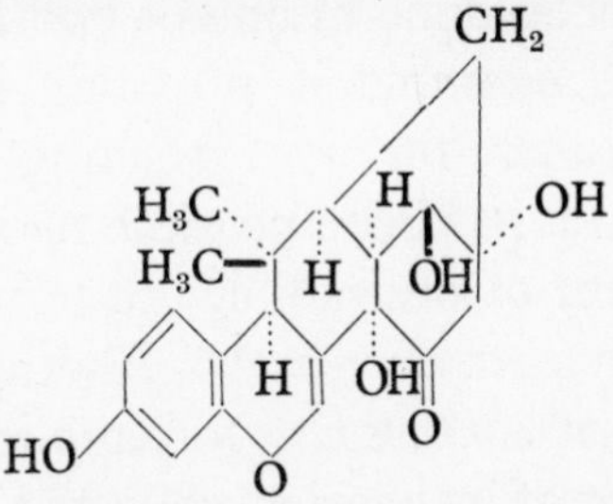

Fig. 25. *Left,* a possible interpretation of the structure of the molecule of stilboestrol. From Emmens, 1962, in *Methods in Hormone Research* (R. I. Dorfman, ed.), **2.** 59–111. (New York: Academic Press). *Right,* the structure of the molecule of miroestrol. From Cain, 1960, *Nature,* **188,** 774.

often be directly correlated with its structure, it is none the less possible for molecules of different structure to have identical or closely similar effects.

Two examples of this may be quoted from the field of oestrogens, the better known being the stilboestrol series of compounds. These are artificial oestrogens, by which is meant that they possess the biological activity of naturally occurring oestrogens, but are chemically different from them, and are known only as products prepared by synthesis in the laboratory. From our present point of view, their interest lies in the fact that they are not steroids at all, and it is still uncertain how they exert their biological effects, although it has been argued that their molecular configuration may resemble that of the natural oestrogens more closely than at first appears (Fig. 25).

The second example of divergence between molecular structure and oestrogenic activity is provided by miroestrol (Fig. 25), a substance that has been extracted from the roots of a Thailand plant known as *Pueraria mirifica*. This substance has markedly oestrogenic properties, so that in one sense it is clearly a naturally occurring oestrogen, but it differs from the oestrogens of vertebrates in that it too, like stilboestrol, is not a steroid. The existence of such a substance in nature, together with the experience afforded by the study of the stilboestrol series of compounds, clearly makes it essential that the molecular basis of the oestrogenic activity of invertebrate extracts should be precisely characterized before any useful interpretation can be placed upon it, but fortunately this has now been done in one or two instances.

One example is provided by the American lobster, *Homarus americanus*, for by extracting some 14,000 g of the eggs of this animal it has been possible to obtain good evidence for the presence in them of oestradiol, the tests employed being in part biological and in part chemical. Another example is found in the starfish, *Pisaster ochraceous*, for application of similar methods to some 6,000 g of its ovaries, collected at the time of spawning, has demonstrated a low level of oestrogenic activity, associated here also with the presence of oestradiol. In this instance, moreover, there was also evidence that progesterone was probably present, which may indicate that this substance is an intermediate stage in the synthesis of oestradiol in the echinoderms, as we have seen it to be in vertebrates.

These facts are admittedly meagre, but they are sufficient to show that oestrogenic steroids are not restricted to vertebrates, and may well have existed before that group appeared. Our consideration of the bile acids, however, has suggested that the establishment of those substances in the vertebrates involved some measure of molecular evolution, and it thus becomes of interest to enquire whether this also applies to the oestrogen molecules, and whether, as posed in our second question, there has been an evolution of oestrogens in response to changing adaptational needs.

Here again our information is still very limited, but oestradiol, oestriol, oestrone, and progesterone have all been identified in ovarian extracts of the toad, *Bufo vulgaris*, which certainly suggests a fundamental similarity in the pathways of oestrogen synthesis in amphibians and mammals. The situation in fish is of particular importance in this connexion, for they represent, despite their particular specializations, an earlier level of vertebrate evolution, and it is thus of great interest that they, too, secrete oestradiol and its related steroids. This hormone has been identified in extracts of the ovaries of the dogfish *Squalus suckleyi*, and of the ray *Torpedo marmorata*, accompanied in the former by oestrone and progesterone, and in the latter by oestriol and progesterone. It is present also in teleosts, for it has been identified in the mature ova of the cod, *Gadus callarias*, together with a smaller concentration of oestrone.

We cannot, of course, assume from this evidence alone that oestradiol is necessarily acting as a sex hormone in these animals, but certain other facts suggest that it may well be doing so. Thus, it is known that its concentration in the ovaries of the cod increases as the ova mature, and its production seems to be particularly characteristic of the female; in the male it is at best only doubtfully identifiable, while neither oestrone nor oestriol have been found in the testes.

Evidence pointing in the same direction comes from the elasmobranchs, for it has been shown that oestradiol has a stimulatory effect upon the oviducts of the dogfish *Scyliorhinus caniculus*. This has been demonstrated by implanting pellets of oestradiol benzoate into the fish so as to provide for a very slow absorption of the hormone over a long period. Fish examined after seven months, when from 11 to 14% of the material had been absorbed, showed increased vascularization of the oviducts, and increased secretion of the horny material which forms the protective 'mermaid's purse' around the fertilized egg. Immature fish did not respond, those that gave this response being those that were already approaching maturity, and this certainly suggests that we are dealing here with a specialized and hormonally-controlled reaction that cannot be evoked in young fish because their tissues have not developed the appropriate sensitivity.

There is, however, a note of warning in the data so far obtained from the cod, for the concentration of oestradiol in its ovaries is much less than that found in mammalian tissues. This could mean that it is not the chief oestrogen in this species, and since other similar, but as yet unidentified, compounds are thought also to be present in extracts of cod ovaries we cannot ignore the possibility that one or other of these may be of physiological importance. The evolutionary history of the oestrogens must, therefore, remain uncertain until the nature and possible functions of these unidentified compounds have been clarified.

One element of the reproductive equipment of the female mammal that merits separate mention is the corpus luteum, which, as we have earlier noted, is an endocrine gland secreting progesterone. This hormone is especially associated with pregnancy, and it is often thought of as being a peculiarly mammalian feature, although the fact that many other vertebrate groups have also evolved viviparity (elasmobranchs and lizards are well-known examples) makes it difficult to be sure if this is really so. However, many authorities doubt whether the ovarian follicles of these lower forms ever give rise to secretory structures after ovulation has taken place, and this certainly suggests that progesterone may indeed function as a hormone only in mammals.

Even if this be so, however, it is obvious that the progesterone molecule certainly does not make its first appearance in that group, for we have found it to be an intermediate stage in the synthesis of other steroid hormones. In this instance, then, the mammalian ovary may have taken into its functional equipment a molecule that was already available in the ovaries of ancestral forms as a metabolic by-product, which is essentially the first of the three possible modes of origin of novelties that we have earlier discussed (p. 17). We must add, nevertheless, that with our present limited information we are far from justified in assuming that progesterone and related compounds are entirely without function in non-mammalian vertebrates, as, indeed, follows from what has been said regarding the unidentified compounds in the ovaries of cod.

An observation bearing upon this issue has emerged from studies of the androgens of fish. Unfortunately very little indeed is known of the androgenic substances present in lower vertebrates, but testosterone has been identified in the testes of the dogfish *Scyliorhinus stellaris*, together with androstenedione, which is believed to be an immediate precursor of testosterone in the mammalian testis. A further similarity between the dogfish and mammal is the presence in the testes of the former of progesterone and oestradiol, so that within this very limited evidence there is at least some suggestion, as there is with the ovary, of similar pathways operating in lower and higher vertebrates.

The possibility that other androgenic steroids may be functional in fish, however, is suggested by the isolation of an unusual androgen from the blood plasma of the male sockeye salmon, *Oncorhynchus nerka*. This androgen, 11-ketosterone, is a derivative of testosterone, and, prior to its discovery in this fish, had been known only as a product of laboratory synthesis. Whether it normally acts as an androgen in this particular species is not known, but it certainly has the capacity to do so, for injection of it into males can evoke changes in form and coloration that are normally developed only at sexual maturity.

It will be obvious that at present we have too little information to permit easy generalization regarding the evolutionary history of the oestrogens and androgens of vertebrates. Nevertheless, it is safe to say that there is no evidence that the extensive reproductive specializations of female mammals have involved any marked evolutionary specialization in their oestrogen equipment. On the contrary, in relying primarily upon oestradiol they are using a molecule that has a history longer than their own, and probably longer than that of the whole of the vertebrate group. In this respect, then, as also in the reliance placed by all vertebrate animals upon cholesterol as their main sterol, we gain an impression of stability in their paths of steroid synthesis, a stability that must have been attained at the beginning of the history of the vertebrates as part of its fundamental pattern of organization. It now remains to see whether similar conclusions are to be drawn from an examination of the history of the corticosteroid hormones.

Evolution and the Corticosteroids

Despite the large number of steroids that have been extracted from adrenocortical tissue, it is well established that the main hormonal products of the tissue in mammals are corticosterone, cortisol (hydrocortisone), and aldosterone, although the proportions in which these are released into the blood stream may vary considerably from species to species. Their functions are complex, but fundamentally they play a major part in the maintenance of that constancy of the internal environment upon which the life of mammalian tissues so closely depends. Among the processes regulated by them are the metabolism of protein and carbohydrate, the transport of electrolytes and water, and the generalized responses of the body to those harmful and exacting conditions in the environment that subject the body to stresses of one kind or another.

As we have already suggested, many of the other steroids extracted from the adrenocortical tissue may be no more than by-products of its biosynthetic activity. Nevertheless, the existence of steroid molecules in such variety would seem to provide effective material for the action of natural selection, and we might on first thoughts expect to find that different types of molecules have been selected at different levels of vertebrate evolution in order to meet more effectively the changing demands set up by the exploitation of new modes of life. The passage from water to dry land, and the development of homoiothermy ('warm-bloodedness'), are but two illustrations of changes that must have profoundly affected the metabolism and the ionic and water relationships of these animals. It is all the more striking, therefore, to find that the lower vertebrates have an adrenocortical secretory pattern that very closely resembles that found in the common laboratory mammals.

The evidence for this has come from two types of procedure, the one *in vivo* and the other *in vitro*. For the former, blood is drawn from the experimental animal, preferably from the adrenal veins, and its corticosteroid content determined, while for the latter a sample of adrenocortical tissue is incubated in a suitable fluid, the steroids produced under these conditions being then collected and identified. In these ways it has been shown that either cortico-sterone, or cortisol, or both, constitute the major corticosteroid output in certain species of birds, reptiles, amphibians, and fish, just as they do in mammals. Aldosterone presents a more difficult problem, for even in the latter group its discovery was delayed because of the small amounts in which it is produced (which, inci-dentally, does not mean that it is unimportant, but that its mole-cule is highly active). There is, however, increasing evidence that this substance, too, is produced at least as far down the vertebrate scale as teleost and elasmobranch fish, although it has not yet been identified in cyclostomes, despite the analysis of no less than 9 litres of blood from the Atlantic hagfish, *Myxine glutinosa*. Cortisol and corticosterone have, nevertheless, been found in this group, both in *Myxine* and also in the Pacific hagfish, *Polistotrema stouti*.

It looks, then, as though the paths of synthesis of the corti-costeroids, like those of the sex steroids, were probably selected and stabilized at a very early stage of vertebrate evolution, al-though not, perhaps, during its protochordate stage, for a study of amphioxus has disclosed no corticosteroids in that animal. This can only mean that the changing metabolic requirements of verte-brates must have been met, as far as these steroids are concerned, by adaptive evolution of their peripheral target organs, rather than of their own molecular structure, and it is not difficult to see a possible reason for this. The action of hormones must presumably depend upon a closely adapted relationship between them and their target cells, enabling them to influence and regulate such elements of cell organization as membrane permeability and enzyme systems. There is thus likely to be strong selection pressure against any change in the molecular structure of the hormones, for this would tend to impair their regulatory activities by interfering with these adaptive relationships, and would thus be highly disadvantageous to the organism. Natural selection would therefore be expected to operate in favour of the stability of the hormonal molecules, and of the metabolic pathways by which they are produced. Adaptive modification of the peripheral target organs, however, would

provide a means of modulating the physiological effects of the hormones in response to new needs, while leaving undisturbed their
fundamental relationships with the cells of the body as a whole.

We lack at present the evidence for adequately testing this line
of argument, but certain observations undoubtedly support the
general proposition of the evolution of target organs. For example,
it is well-known that the highly permeable gills of fish make an
important contribution to the exchange of ions and water between
the animal and the external medium, sea-water or fresh water as
the case may be, and evidence that these are under the control of
corticosteroids comes from experiments in which the injection of
these substances has been shown to promote increased outflow of
sodium from the gills. Another example comes from frogs, for
here there is evidence that removal of the adrenal glands (adrenalectomy) results in an increased loss of sodium through the highly
permeable skin. Both of these illustrations show how highly
specialized responses, peculiar to particular groups, may be mediated by hormonal mechanisms, without, as far as we are aware, any
concomitant specialization of the hormonal molecules concerned.
The specialization lies in the relevant target cells, located in these
instances in the gills and the skin respectively, and constituting an
effector mechanism that is not present in that particular form in
mammals.

One other example, and a particularly striking one, is provided
by the very different response to marine conditions given by birds,
on the one hand, and mammals, on the other. It is only too well
known that shipwrecked mariners cannot maintain life by drinking
sea-water. This is because they absorb large amounts of salts in
doing this, and can only remove these salts by excreting even more
water than they have taken in; the result is necessarily a progressive dehydration.

Now marine birds may be out of reach of fresh water for long
periods of time. Whether they are thus driven to drink sea-water
is not certain, for they can take in much moisture with their food,
but it is quite certain that they can readily drink it under laboratory
conditions, and can survive unharmed. This they are able to do

because they possess specialized glands called the nasal glands (Fig. 26), paired structures that lie above the eye, and are so large in some marine species that they give rise to prominent grooves in the wall of the skull. The ingestion of sea-water is followed by an increased output of fluid from this gland, and droplets of secretion appear on the beak, where their ducts open to the outside. The

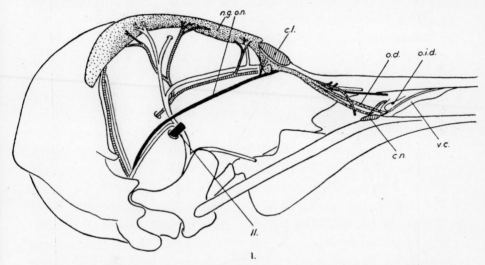

Fig. 26. Diagram of a dissection of the head of an oyster-catcher, showing the nasal gland and its ducts, and the associated blood vessels. *c.l.*, cut end of lachrymal bone; *c.n.*, cut end of nasal bone; *n.g.*, nasal gland; *o.d.*, outer duct; *o.i.d.*, opening of inner duct on nasal septum; *o.n.*, ophthalmic nerve; *v.c.*, vestibular concha; *II*, optic nerve. From Marples, 1932, *Proc. zool. Soc. Lond.*, 829–844.

bird shakes off these 'avian dew-drops', and in so doing removes from its body a fluid that contains a higher salt content than either the blood plasma or the urine. As a result, it can benefit from the drinking of sea-water by being able to retain some of the water while readily discarding the surplus salts.

From our present point of view the interest of this phenomenon lies in evidence that the nasal glands are under the control of the corticosteroids. The evidence comes from experiments on domestic ducks (Fig. 27), which have shown that the secretory activity of the glands can be reduced by adrenalectomy, and can be restored to a normal level in adrenalectomized ducks by injecting them with corticosteroids. This, then, would seem to be another example of an adaptive response, peculiar to a particular group of vertebrates, and dependent upon the specialized properties of an organ that is

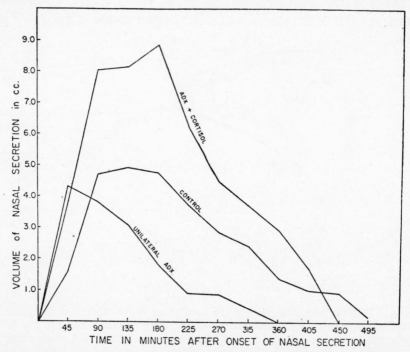

Fig. 27. Effects of adrenalectomy and cortisol administration on the secretory activity of the nasal gland of the domestic duck, following the introduction into the stomach of 20 ml. of 20% sodium chloride solution. *Middle curve,* normal control animals; *lower curve,* animals with one adrenal gland removed, showing reduced activity; *upper curve,* animal with both adrenal glands removed, but receiving cortisol, showing that secretory activity is fully restored by treatment with the hormone. From Phillips *et al.,* 1961, *Endocrinology,* **69,** 958–969.

equally peculiar to the group. Natural selection has determined the evolution of the nasal glands, and in so doing has established a close relationship between them and an already existing hormone or hormones. The latter, however, remain unaltered, a situation that, on our above argument, must be in itself of the greatest adaptive advantage, for it leaves the other functions of those hormones undisturbed.

3 The Hormones of the Thyroid Gland

'Dear me,' said Mr. Grewgious, peeping in, 'it's like looking down the throat of Old Time.'
Charles Dickens: *Edwin Drood*

The Biosynthesis of the Thyroid Hormones

THE secretory activity of the thyroid gland depends upon the properties of tyrosine (Fig. 30). This is a phenolic amino acid, with a molecular structure based upon a six-carbon ring to which are attached a hydroxyl group and a side chain, the latter consisting of another amino acid, alanine. Tyrosine plays an important part in several biosynthetic pathways, for it is the source of the brown or black pigments called melanins, which arise from it as a result of its oxidation, while it is also a precursor of adrenaline and noradrenaline (p. 26), two substances that are chemically related to catechol, and that belong to a group of compounds known as catecholamines.

Noradrenaline and adrenaline (Fig. 28), the so-called catechol hormones, are secreted by the chromaffin tissue of vertebrates, but, as we have noted, they are not confined to that group. Both have been extracted from the central nervous system of earthworms, and they are also known to be present in many insects, although their functions in these animals are unknown. There is also some evidence that other invertebrates may synthesize closely related substances; the salivary gland of the common octopus, for example, contains octopamine, a catechol derivative that can be transformed into noradrenaline by ultraviolet irradiation. It would seem, then, that here, as with the steroid hormones, the vertebrates may be making use of a biosynthetic pathway that has also been established in other groups, and that may well have been present in their

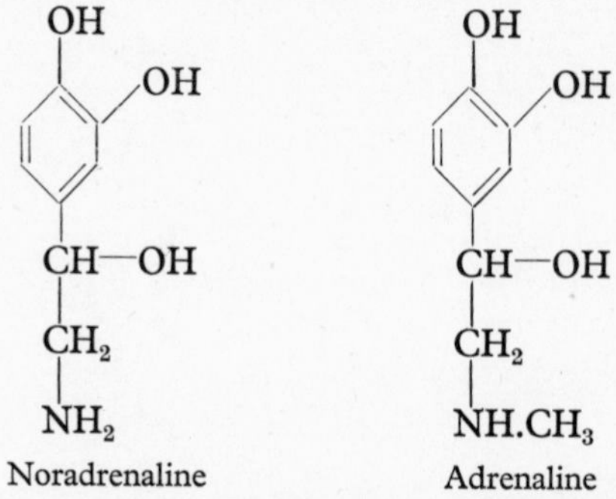

Fig. 28.   Molecular structure of the catechol hormones.

immediate ancestors, although we have no satisfactory information on this point; indeed, tests carried out on the protochordate amphioxus have failed to give any clear indication of the presence of catecholamines in that animal.

The involvement of tyrosine in the synthesis of the thyroid hormones depends upon its capacity for combining with free iodine, which can become attached to the phenol ring at the C_3 and C_5 positions, and which is then said to be organically bound. The investigation of this process has been greatly aided by the employment of radioactive iodine (I^{131}) in the techniques of autoradiography, chromatography, and electrophoresis, for this has made possible a close study of the iodine metabolism of the thyroid gland, including the identification and quantitative determination of micro-quantities of its products.

These techniques are too elaborate to be described here in any detail, but they can be said to depend in general upon the administration of a small dose (called a tracer dose) of radioactive iodide to the experimental animals, either by injection or, in the case of aquatic forms, by solution in the water surrounding them. If iodine binding is taking place the resulting compounds will be identifiable, even in very minute quantities, by virtue of their radioactivity, and they are said to be 'labelled' by radioiodine.

If their identification is to be carried out by paper chromatography, extracts are prepared from the appropriate tissues, and

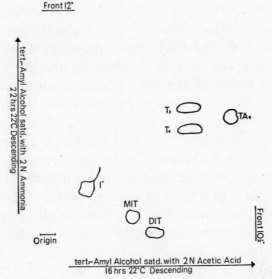

Fig. 29. The use of two-dimensional chromatography to separate iodide (I), MIT, DIT, T_3, T_4 (cf. Fig. 30), and TA_4 (cf. Fig. 31). The initial spot was placed at the bottom left-hand corner; the direction of flow of the two solvents is indicated by arrows.

small drops of these extracts are placed upon filter paper. Solvents are then applied to the paper when it is in a vertical position, and these separate the various components of the drops by moving them over the paper at different rates. As a result, the contents of each drop are distributed in a characteristic pattern of spots. One such solvent may be adequate for this purpose (one-dimensional chromatography), or it may be advantageous to use two in succession (Fig. 29), applied so that the substances are moved first in one direction and then in another at right angles to it (two-dimensional chromatography). In either case the spots that contain bound radioiodine will be recognizable by their radioactivity, and the substances carrying the iodine can then be identified by comparing their positions with the distribution of spots of known compounds after they have been treated with similar solvents. Electrophoresis is somewhat similar in its effects, in so far as this also involves the movement of substances at characteristic rates over filter paper, but in this instance the movement is brought about by the application to the paper of an electric potential.

These methods make it possible to establish the presence within particular tissues of remarkably small quantities of iodinated compounds, and they can be supplemented by the use of autoradiography, which allows of the very precise localization within the body of iodinated compounds formed after the administration of radioiodine. This technique involves preparing sections of the tissues, mounting them on slides, and applying a photographic film to them. The film is exposed for a suitable period, and is then developed, whereupon the sites of accumulation of radioiodine will be visible on it as images of reduced silver. The histological techniques may be expected to dissolve out all of the inorganic iodine, so that these sites will indicate the areas in which it has been organically bound.

As a result of these procedures, and arising out of the earlier studies of Kendall and of Harington, we can speak with some precision of the course of events leading to the production of the thyroid hormones. The essential facts are that the secretory epithelium of the thyroid gland traps iodide from the circulating blood, and does so with such efficiency that if a tracer dose of radioiodide is injected into a rat the gland may have taken up as much as 20% of the dose within 16 hours, a remarkable figure having regard to the very small size of the organ. Within the cells the iodide is rapidly oxidized to free iodine through the agency of an appropriate enzyme system, and then becomes bound to tyrosine. This is not present as a free amino acid, but as part of the molecular structure of thyroglobulin, a protein that contains bound carbohydrate, and that belongs to the group of substances called glycoproteins (p. 104). Thyroglobulin forms the major part of the so-called thyroid colloid, which, stored within the follicles of the gland, is a characteristic feature of its histological structure. It is also present as droplets within the epithelial cells that secrete it, and it is probably within these rather than within the mass of stored colloid that the iodinating reactions take place.

The iodinated tyrosine molecules (Fig. 30) are 3-mono-iodo-tyrosine (MIT for short), and 3,5-di-iodotyrosine (DIT), so named

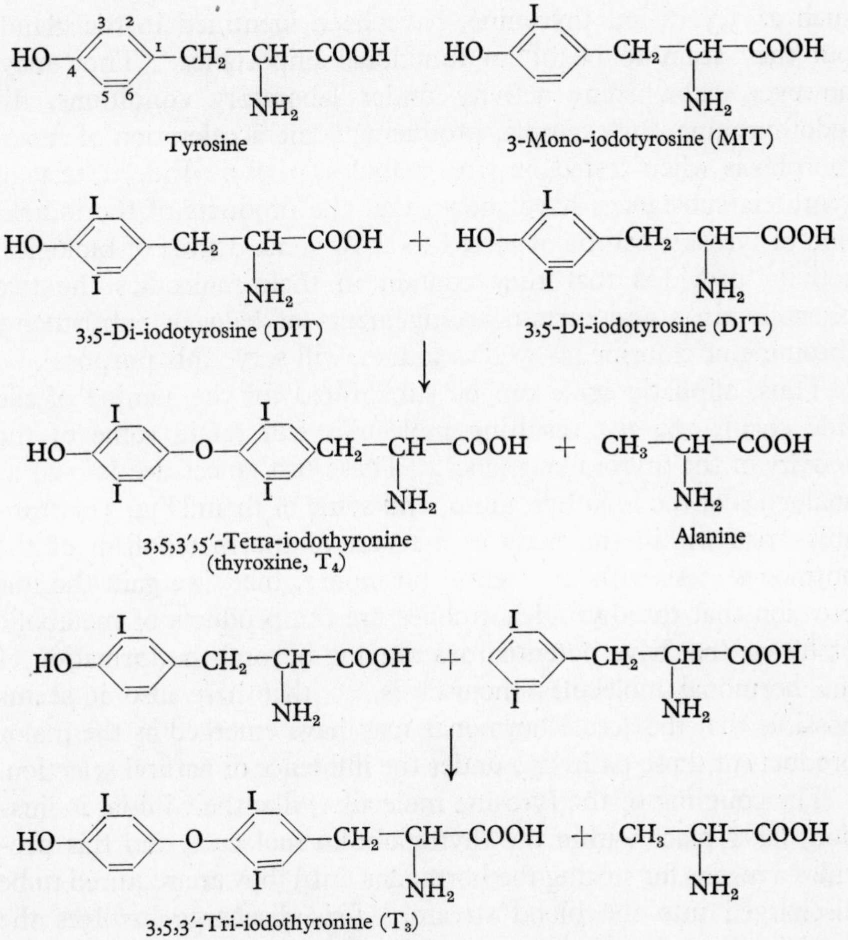

Fig. 30. The iodination of tyrosine, and the formation of the hormones of the thyroid gland by coupling of the iodotyrosine molecules.

according to whether they contain one or two iodine substitutions. They are not themselves the hormones, for they lack biological activity, and the hormonal synthesis has to be completed by their condensation in pairs, with the loss of a single alanine residue. This results in the formation of two compounds called 3,5,3'-tri-iodothyronine (T_3) and 3,5,3',5'-tetra-iodothyronine (T_4, thyroxine), and these are regarded as the thyroid hormones, for they are biologically active and are known to be released into the blood.

Other condensation products are theoretically possible, and some, such as 3,3'-di-iodothyronine, have been identified in the gland, but they seem to be of no functional importance. They may, however, show some activity under laboratory conditions, di-iodothyronine, for example, producing some acceleration of meta-morphosis when tested on frog tadpoles (p. 91). Indeed, tests of synthetic substances have shown that the products of the iodina-tion of tyrosine can be expected to show some degree of biological activity provided that they contain in their molecules the two phenolic rings and certain arrangements of halogen substituents (bromine or chlorine, as well as iodine, will serve this purpose).

Thus, aliphatic acids can be substituted for the alanine of the side chain, and the resulting molecules will retain some of the activity of the thyroid hormones. These substances are known as analogues of the iodothyronines, and some of them (Fig. 31) prob-ably arise within the body as a result of the metabolism of the hormones. As with the steroid hormones, then, we gain the im-pression that the thyroid hormones are the products of metabolic pathways that have potentialities ranging beyond the formation of the hormonal molecules themselves, so that here also it seems possible that the actual hormones may have emerged as the major products of those pathways under the influence of natural selection.

The coupling of the tyrosine molecules, like their initial iodina-tion, takes place within the thyroglobulin molecule, and this pro-vides a means for storing the hormones until they are required to be discharged into the blood stream. This discharge involves the participation of two enzymes. One of these is a protease, which breaks down the thyroglobulin and thus releases the iodinated tyrosine and thyronine residues, while the other is a deiodinase, which specifically removes the iodine from the tyrosines but leaves the thyronines untouched. As a result of this remarkable specialization, the hormonal molecules are released into the circulation, while the tyrosines and their liberated iodine are retained within the gland to take part in another cycle of biosynthesis. It is clear, then, that we are dealing here with a highly specialized

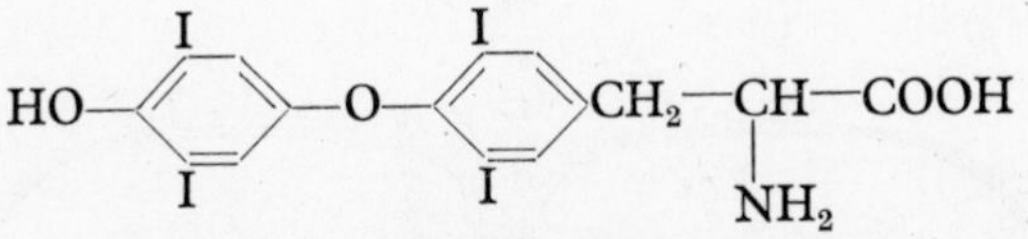

Thyroxine (T$_4$)

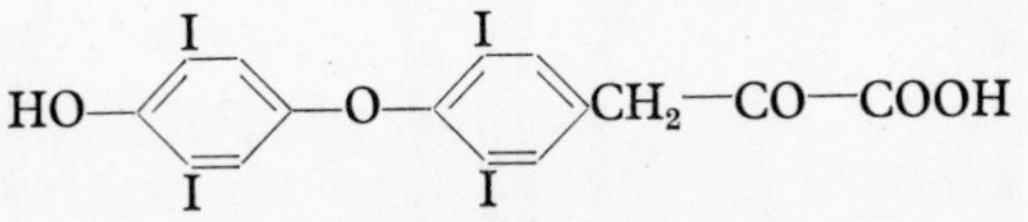

3,5,3′,5′-Thyropyruvic acid (TP$_4$)

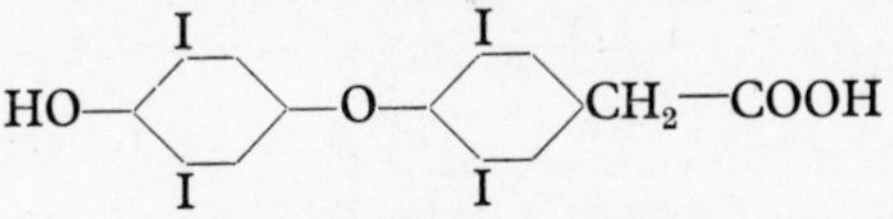

3,5,3′,5′-Thyroacetic acid (TA$_4$)

Fig. 31. Molecular structure of thyroxine and two of its analogues.

tissue equipped to carry out a complex but well-organized sequence of chemical events.

It is difficult to conceive of these events arising for the first time in an already perfected state, and it would seem altogether more likely that they must be the product of a long evolutionary history. Nevertheless, we find not only that the histological organization of the thyroid gland is remarkably uniform throughout the vertebrates, down to and including the adult cyclostomes, but that this uniformity applies also to the pattern of its iodine metabolism. In species from all of the main groups, cyclostomes, fish, amphibians, reptiles, and birds, the production of thyroxine and 3,5,3′-tri-iodothyronine has been demonstrated, and, what is more remarkable, it has been shown that the typical pattern of thyroidal biosynthesis is already established in the endostyle of the ammocoete larva of the lamprey.

This organ lies beneath the pharynx as a hollow tubular structure, very different in appearance from the follicular thyroid gland of the adult. Autoradiography has clearly demonstrated, however, that parts of its specialized epithelium (Fig. 32) are able to bind iodine into a secretory product that is discharged into the

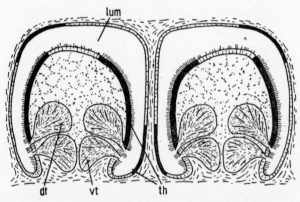

Fig. 32. Diagram of a transverse section of the endostyle of an ammocoete larva (cf. Fig. 10). The chief regions of iodine binding, as revealed by auto-radiography, are shown in black. *dt.*, dorsal glandular tract; *lum.*, lumen of endostyle; *th.*, iodine-binding epithelium; *vt.*, ventral glandular tract. From Barrington, 1962, *Experientia*, **18**, 201–210.

cavity of the endostyle and passes out from it into the pharynx. There is some reason for believing that it is then carried with the ingested food material into the intestine, where it can presumably be digested and absorbed. Extracts of the endostyle have been shown by paper chromatography to contain 3-mono-iodotyrosine, 3,5-di-iodotyrosine, and the two hormones, while hormonally bound iodine has been found in the blood, all of which suggests that the hormones may well be of biological importance in lamprey larvae, although the functions that they fulfil are still unknown. What is quite clear, however, is that the endostyle at this stage of evolution has all the essential features of the biosynthetic capacity of the thyroid gland, although, as might be expected, its capacity for trapping iodide is much feebler than that of the mammalian thyroid, while biosynthesis is known to proceed in it at a comparatively slow rate. Evidently, then, our search for evidence relating to the origin of thyroidal biosynthesis and of the thyroid hormones must be extended to include also the invertebrate animals.

Iodine Binding in Invertebrates

Facts of central importance in any consideration of the origin of the thyroid hormones are, first, that iodine is comparatively abundant in the sea, where there may be as much as 50 micrograms per litre, compared with the 1 microgram per litre of rain-water, and second, that many marine animals maintain a high concentration of the element within their body or in its secretions. Examples of this are sponges, which may contain up to 2·35%, the horny skeletons of the gorgonid coelenterates, which contain up to 10%, the calcareous tubes of the polychaete *Serpula columbrana*, with 0·30%, and the cuticle of the horse-clam, with 0·298%. These values are surprisingly high, for comparable estimates of the iodine content of thyroid glands, determined by the same chemical procedure, have given figures ranging from 0·096% for the dog to 1·160% for large dogfish.

It is only within the last few years, however, that it has been appreciated that much of this iodine may be present in organically bound form. For example, chromatography of extracts of the gorgonid *Eunicella*, after immersion of the animals in sea-water containing radioiodide, has shown that organically bound radioiodine is present, much of it as 3-mono-iodotyrosine, together with rather less as 3,5-di-iodotyrosine. However, although the concentrations of these two substances range from 8 to 12%, no more than trace quantities of thyroxine and 3,5,3′-tri-iodothyronine have been identified, representing concentrations of the order of only 0·1–0·2%. Moreover, in order to obtain these iodinated compounds in a free state it is necessary to hydrolyse the skeletal axis by boiling in 6N caustic soda for as long as 18 hours, in marked contrast to the enzymatic hydrolysis by trypsin, which is adequate to release the corresponding compounds from the thyroglobulin of thyroid gland extracts.

There are, then, important differences between the iodination that goes on in *Eunicella* and the processes that are characteristic of the thyroid gland. In the former, only minute quantities of biologically active compounds are produced, and then in a form that is so firmly bound that it can hardly be available for use within the organism, whereas the thyroid gland is able to manufacture large quantities of the iodothyronines within protein molecules, from which they are readily freed under biological conditions. It is thought that the explanation of these differences may be that the tyrosine molecules that take up iodine in *Eunicella* form component parts of what are called scleroproteins, or structural proteins. It is these that form the protein basis of skeletal material and protective secretions, and because of this they are characterized by their very tough and fibrous nature, and by their resistance to enzymatic digestion. The suggestion is that iodine binding in *Eunicella* is not a specialized process, evolved as a secretory adaptation like the iodine binding of the thyroid gland, but is simply a consequence of the random iodination of tyrosine residues that happen to be present in the skeleton. This could account for the fact that only minute quantities of the iodinated thyronines are formed, for the tyrosine residues may be thought of as distributed through the fibrous molecules of the structural proteins in a manner that offers little opportunity for them to become coupled.

It seems likely that this interpretation may be applicable to other cases of iodination of skeletal material in invertebrates, an example of which is provided by molluscs, for autoradiograms have shown that considerable amounts of radioactive iodine collect over the surface of the shell and body of these animals. It has been suggested that this may be largely a result of simple adsorption from the radioactive sea-water, but it is doubtful whether this could account completely for the accumulation of the iodine, for there is some evidence that this is particularly associated with the newly formed parts of the shell. These are the regions where fresh scleroprotein is being synthesized, and it seems possible, therefore, that iodine may become organically bound to this material. Moreover, paper chromatography has clearly shown the presence of 3-mono-iodotyrosine in *Mytilus*, although there are no more than traces of 3,5-di-iodotyrosine, and no evidence at all for the presence of the iodothyronines.

We cannot safely generalize from these data until a much wider range of species has been studied in these ways, but we know enough to suspect that the background of the evolution of the thyroidal hormones bears a certain resemblance to the situation that we have discussed in connexion with the steroid hormones, and yet also shows some differences. The fundamental pathways of steroid biosynthesis seem to be widespread, if not universal, in living organisms, and they seem to constitute from the beginning a well-defined feature of the metabolism of cells. The organic binding of iodine to form iodotyrosines is also widespread, but an important difference is that the formation of iodothyronines is much more restricted in its incidence, and this suggests that the process as a whole has been subjected to a great deal of adaptive evolution. It seems likely, for example, that the molecular structure of thyroglobulin may be such as to facilitate the coupling of its tyrosine residues, and it may also be that this coupling is further aided in the thyroid gland by an appropriate enzyme system. Unfortunately, our information is still too limited for us to be able to judge the course of this evolution, and the interpretation of the facts that are available is a matter of some disagreement. In the hope, therefore, of achieving further clarification of these issues, and of the possible relationships between the random binding of iodine and the highly organized process of thyroidal biosynthesis, much attention has been focused upon the Protochordata, particularly in view of the known relationship of the endostyle with the thyroid gland (p. 23).

Iodine Binding in the Protochordata

Included in the Subphylum Hemichordata is a group that forms the Class Enteropneusta and is represented by *Saccoglossus*. The enteropneusts are worm-like animals that are found burrowing in sand, mud, or shell-gravel between and below the tide marks, and it is probably fair to say that the only characteristic of the adults that carries strong conviction as a chordate feature is the structure of the gill slits, which strikingly resembles that of the developing gills of the Tunicata and of amphioxus. It is possible to discern in the structure of the nervous system of the collar region some indication of the dorsal tubular nerve cord of other chordates, but the suggestion that the stomochord, a small evagination of the alimentary canal, is homologous with the notochord has failed to win general acceptance. Moreover, the hemichordates have no trace of an endostyle. It cannot be denied, however, that the tornaria larva of certain enteropneusts bears a striking resemblance to the dipleurula larva of echinoderms, and, even if the animals are excluded from the Phylum Chordata, they can reasonably be regarded as closely related both to them and also to the echinoderms, which are generally held to be the invertebrates that lie closest to the ancestry of that Phylum.

Enteropneusts secrete an abundance of mucus-like material from their body surface, and it seems that some of this is used for entangling food (Fig. 16), and some for making a temporary lining to their burrows. So little is known of the general biology of these animals, however, that it is difficult to speak with much assurance of these matters, but it is at least certain that iodine does become organically bound to some of this secretion. This can be detected in autoradiograms of *Saccoglossus* if the animals are maintained for some 48 hours in sea-water containing radioactive iodide, and the autoradiograms further show that under these laboratory conditions some of the iodinated secretion is passed forwards towards the mouth and may even enter the alimentary canal.

It would, of course, be attractive to suppose, on the basis of this evidence, that enteropneusts are able to synthesize and to ingest some form of thyroidal product, but chromatographic analysis has so far given no support to this possibility. All that is revealed on paper chromatograms is iodide and 3-mono-iodotyrosine (Fig. 33), so that although some iodination of tyrosine is certainly taking place, the process stops at an early stage. It follows from this that even in a protochordate the mere presence of organically bound iodine is no evidence for the occurrence of the complete sequence of reactions involved in thyroidal biosynthesis. Moreover, the distribution of bound iodine in autoradiograms indicates

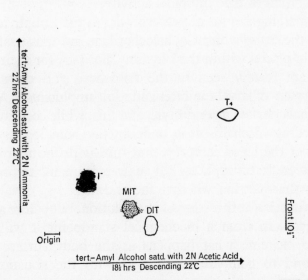

Fig. 33. The use of two-dimensional chromatography to show the formation of MIT by *Saccoglossus horsti*. The two black areas show the presence of radioactive iodine (cf. Fig. 29). From Barrington and Thorpe, 1963, *Gen. comp. Endocrin.*, **3**, 166–175.

that much of the binding takes place when the secretion has been discharged from the cells of the surface epithelium into the surrounding water, rather than within the cells themselves. This suggests that the binding may not be primarily a metabolic process at all, but a consequence of iodine being randomly bound to tyrosine residues present in the discharged secretion, a situation closely analogous to the iodination of scleroproteins. Presumably there must be some oxidizing system present to convert the iodide into iodine, but such systems are common enough in organisms, and there is no reason to suppose that its presence need be in any

way an adaptation related to iodine binding.   There is no justification, then, for regarding the Enteropneusta as being engaged in
thyroidal biosynthesis.   The situation that they present, however,
is none the less an interesting one, for at least it demonstrates the
possibility of animals ingesting iodinated products that happen to
be formed by chance over their body surface, and we shall see
that this might conceivably have played a part of some importance
in the evolution of true thyroidal activity.

The remaining groups of protochordates, the Subphylum Tunicata, and the Subphylum Cephalochordata, are universally agreed
to be justly placed within the Phylum Chordata, for their chordate
affinities are readily seen in the notochord and dorsal tubular
nervous system of larval tunicates and adult amphioxus.   Moreover,
these animals possess an endostyle, and this, while constituting part
of the feeding mechanism, is undoubtedly homologous with the
endostyle of the larval lamprey, and thus with the thyroid gland.
We have seen that morphological analysis is unable to provide any
answer to the question whether the endostyle has developed any
thyroidal function at this stage of its evolution, but before approaching the problem from a biochemical standpoint it will be con-
venient to examine what happens at the body surface of these
animals, and to compare the results with the situation in the
Enteropneusta.

A species that has been closely studied from the point of view
of iodine binding is *Ciona intestinalis*, a member of the group of
sessile tunicates that constitute the Class Ascidacea.   Its body is
covered with the thick tunic that gives the name to the whole
Subphylum, and that is unique among animals in being composed
largely of cellulose.   A protein component is also present, however,
for cells that migrate through this tunic accumulate at its surface
and there secrete a protein layer that presumably serves as a protective covering.   By analogy with the invertebrates that we have
already discussed, this would seem to be a potential site of iodine
binding, and autoradiograms do, in fact, show that when *Ciona* is
immersed in radioiodinated sea-water a considerable amount of
bound iodine accumulates in this surface layer.   Whether this is a

result of random binding, as in the examples that we have already discussed, is not yet clear, but chromatographic studies have shown that the results are certainly more complex than those observed in *Saccoglossus*, for both 3-mono-iodotyrosine and 3,5-diiodotyrosine are formed, together with a number of other iodinated compounds. The results seem to be influenced by the conditions in which the animals have been maintained, and by the temperature to which they are adapted, but there is evidence that thyroid hormones can be formed in some circumstances. It appears, then, that iodine binding in the tunic may result in the production of biologically active compounds, although the full significance of this cannot be judged on the evidence so far obtained.

Fortunately, more clear-cut evidence has been obtained from studies of the endostyle. As we have seen, this organ is not present in the Hemichordata, but is well developed both in the Tunicata and in amphioxus, as a groove running along the length of the large pharynx. It consists of ciliated and secretory cells, the latter arranged in glandular tracts that closely resemble those of the endostyle of the ammocoete larva. At the protochordate level of evolution its function is primarily alimentary, for it produces a mucous secretion that is swept up the sides of the pharynx and traps food particles contained in the current of water passing through that organ. This secretion, with the accumulated food material, is then driven by cilia along the dorsal wall of the pharynx and on into the intestine.

Having regard to the known thyroidal activity of the endostyle in the ammocoete larva, it is of great interest that autoradiography of animals that have been maintained in radioiodinated sea-water clearly demonstrates the presence of bound iodine in parts of the epithelium of the organ, both in tunicates and in amphioxus (Figs. 34, 35). Just as in the ammocoete, no binding takes place in the glandular tracts; instead, the bound iodine is localized in clearly defined groups of cells situated immediately above the tracts, in a position similar in principle to that of the epithelium in which much of the iodine binding takes place in the ammocoete's endostyle. This localization in itself implies that we are dealing here with a specialized function of a limited region of the epithelium, rather than with mere random binding, and this in its turn suggests that the endostyle may have developed a truly thyroidal type of iodine metabolism.

Paper chromatographic studies of extracts of whole bodies of

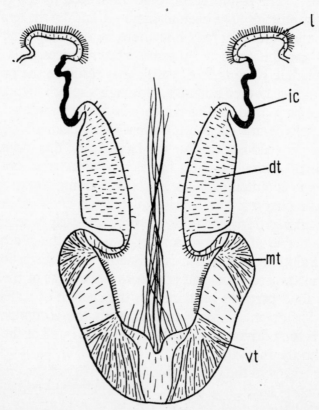

Fig. 34. Diagram of a transverse section of the endostyle of Ciona. *dt.*, *mt.*, *vt.*, dorsal, median, and ventral glandular tracts; *ic.*, iodination centres; l., lip of endostyle. × 300. From Barrington, 1962. *Experientia*, **18**, 201–210.

amphioxus, after the usual immersion in radioiodinated sea-water, go a long way to confirm this, for they show the presence of mono-iodotyrosine, 3,5-di-iodotyrosine, 3,5,3′-tri-iodothyronine, and thyroxine, together with the acetic acid analogues of the hormones. This spectrum of compounds clearly indicates the occurrence of typical thyroidal biosynthesis. Moreover, these substances, or at least the tyrosines and the two hormones, have been identified both in extracts of the endostylar region of the pharynx and also in the remainder of the soft tissues, although with a greater concentration in the former. This suggests that the endostyle plays a leading

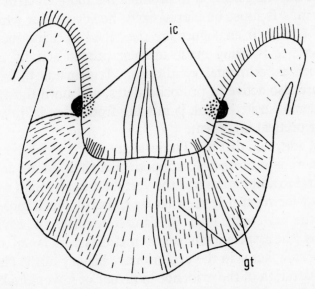

Fig. 35. Diagram of a transverse section of the endostyle of *Branchiostoma* (amphioxus). *ic.*, iodination centres; *gt.*, glandular tracts. × 500. From Barrington, 1962. *Experientia*, **18**, 201–210.

part in their formation, but that other tissues may also share in this, a suggestion that carries the further interesting implication that the localization of thyroidal properties in the endostyle (and hence in the thyroid gland) may be a consequence of the later restriction to a specific organ of synthetic capacities that were originally more widespread in the tissues of early chordates.

It is this that gives particular interest to the occurrence of iodine binding in the tunic of ascidians, for surface binding might constitute a step in the evolution of the thyroidal biosynthesis of higher chordates. The argument is based upon the supposition that if a tissue such as the tunic is able to form biologically active substances, these might become metabolically available to the organism, perhaps as a result of their breakdown within the tissue, or perhaps by the ingestion of fragments shed from the body surface, just as *Saccoglossus* ingests its iodinated secretion. If these substances then proved to be of advantage to the species concerned, even though they were initially available only in trace quantities, it would then be possible for natural selection to promote the more efficient production of them. It must be emphasized, however, that when iodothyronines and their analogues are described as being biologically active, reference is being made to their proven activity in vertebrates under experimental conditions. It remains to be shown that they are also active in protochordates, and until this has actually been demonstrated a link is missing from what is, in any case, a highly theoretical argument.

We must add, too, that the Tunicata are very specialized animals, and that there is no reason to suppose that their adults are in any way ancestral to amphioxus and the vertebrates, although a case can be made out for regarding their larvae as being much more closely related to the vertebrate line. This case involves the assumption that neoteny (the association of sexual maturity with larval organization) has been a factor in the evolutionary history of the chordates, but a consideration of the evidence in favour of it would take us too far afield. In any case, it seems wiser at this stage to regard the occurrence of iodine binding in the ascidian tunic as being no more than a suggestion of the way in which events might have proceeded in early forerunners of the vertebrates. Our knowledge of the mode of origin of the latter from protochordates is unlikely ever to be more than fragmentary, for the protochordates surviving today are but highly specialized members of what must have been originally a much more extensive fauna. It would be going altogether too far, therefore, to claim to see anything in the nature of a clear-cut evolutionary sequence in the various types of iodine binding that have at present been found in the Protochordata.

The importance of the endostyle as a centre of iodine binding in these animals is, however, quite clear, at least as far as amphioxus is concerned. The evidence from *Ciona* is not so complete, although iodinated compounds are present in extracts of its endostyle, while autoradiograms, as we have seen, also show that some form of bound iodine is certainly present in that organ. Probably, then, the endostyle in this animal has at least something of the thyroidal properties of the endostyle of amphioxus, and it may well be asked why this particular organ should have come into prominence in this way. We can only guess at the answer, of course, but it is possible to see that the central role of the endostyle in ciliary feeding might make it well suited for the manufacture of biologically valuable compounds that could then be added to the food cord with reasonable assurance of their eventual absorption by the alimentary canal. Indeed, it is possible that thyroidal biosynthesis may have arisen from the beginning as a by-product of the secretory activity of the endostyle, and that the iodine-binding activity of the body surfaces of the protochordates had no direct influence upon the history of the thyroid gland.

We have now carried our analysis to a point at which we may draw some conclusions from the evidence obtained from these studies of the protochordates. It is apparent that the thyroidal capacity of the endostyle of the ammocoete larva is not something that appears as an entirely new development in the vertebrates. On the contrary, the organic binding of iodine is widespread in the protochordates, and has been elaborated in amphioxus to full thyroidal status, as far as we may judge from the substances produced. It is possible that the Tunicata stand somewhere between the Hemichordata and amphioxus in the complexity of the iodinated compounds that they form, although this remains uncertain. Such a biochemical situation would, however, be fully conformable with the respective evolutionary status of the three groups as reflected in their anatomical organization, for the Cephalochordata are much closer to the vertebrate plan of structure than are the Tunicata, while the connexion of the Enteropneusta with the vertebrates is at best somewhat tenuous. It may be, then, that biochemical evolution may eventually prove to have paralleled morphological evolution in this respect.

As regards the history of the endostyle, it will be noticed that these observations show that this organ did not become completely transformed into a thyroid gland at one particular stage of its evolution. What seems to have happened is that groups of its cells developed some degree of thyroidal capacity while the rest of the organ retained its old function as part of the feeding mechanism, so that two distinct functions, thyroidal and alimentary, were being carried on at the same time. Indeed, this applies not only to the protochordates but also to the ammocoete larva, for even in the endostyle of that animal, where thyroidal biosynthesis is much more extensively developed than it is in the endostyle of amphioxus, the glandular tracts do not take part in iodine binding.

We may regard this as an example of the principle of mosaic evolution, a term first introduced to describe the way in which morphological transformation takes place when one type of organization is giving rise to another. In such circumstances it is well known that the various parts of the body do not all change at the same rate, so that *Archaeopteryx*, for example, retained a reptilian tail after it had developed the feathers of a bird, and claws after it had developed wings. Transitional stages of evolution are thus represented by animals that are mosaics of old and new, and the same is evidently true of the endostyle.

Evolution and the Thyroid Hormones

Our consideration of the evolution of the steroid hormones led us to visualize this as being a result of the natural selection of certain products and certain metabolic pathways out of the wide spectrum of products that living protoplasm seems to be so readily able to form. By contrast, the evolution of the thyroid hormones is less easy to visualize, and two interpretations have, in fact, been put forward. One of these suggests that there is no evolutionary relationship at all between the random formation of metabolically inert iodinated compounds within the molecules of scleroproteins and the formation of metabolically active compounds within the thyroglobulin molecule. The question of the mode of origin of the latter compounds is thus left unanswered, except in so far as it is ascribed to the iodine-binding capacity of a ubiquitous amino acid, and the existence of iodinated scleroproteins in invertebrate animals is regarded as no more than an irrelevant consequence of that capacity.

The other interpretation (p. 83) suggests that there may be a direct relationship between the two types of iodination, that thyroxine formed under certain conditions by scleroproteins might have become metabolically available, perhaps by ingestion or breakdown of the iodinated material, and that this could have led to the development of more efficient iodination mechanisms within the endostyle and thyroid gland, always, of course, under the influence of natural selection.

It is arguable that, from the standpoint of evolutionary theory, there is no real difference of principle between these two viewpoints, for in both cases thyroidal biosynthesis must ultimately have evolved out of the capacity of tyrosine to take up iodine, and, in so doing, to form biologically active compounds. Essentially this represents the first of the three possibilities discussed earlier (p. 17), the evolution of novelties out of by-products, and it may be felt to be a matter of detail (although admittedly a very interesting one) whether the initial production of these compounds was localized in skeletal and protective products of the body surface, or in one or other of the internal tissues. It would be unprofitable now to discuss this particular matter any further, and we may turn instead to consider the implications of the very evident fact that the pathways of thyroidal biosynthesis, whatever may have been the cause of their inception, were being established within the endostyle during the protochordate stage of evolution. Their fundamental features, including the production of the iodinated thyronines, are, in consequence, fully developed at the very beginning of vertebrate evolution, and thereafter there has been no change in the nature and structure of the hormonal molecules.

We arrived at similar conclusions for the steroid hormones, but with less certainty, and leaving open the possibility that there may have been some diminution in the spectrum of steroid hormonal molecules during vertebrate history. In principle, however, both sets of hormones, steroid and thyroidal, present us with the problem

D

of determining how the widely varying adaptive needs of vertebrates could have been adequately satisfied by hormones in which
evolutionary change has been minimal or non-existent.   In our
review of the steroid hormones, and particularly those of the
adrenocortical tissue, we have seen evidence that these needs have
been met with adaptive evolution of the target tissues.   In dealing
now with the functions of the thyroid hormones we shall be led
to a similar conclusion, and by evidence of somewhat greater
precision.

One of the best-known effects of the thyroid hormones is their
influence upon the basal metabolic rate of mammals.   It is well
established that injection of thyroid extracts into these animals will
evoke a marked increase in oxygen consumption, while it has been
known since 1895 that human patients suffering from myxoedema
(p. 4) have an abnormally low metabolic rate.   Associated with
this effect is the involvement of the thyroid hormones in the regulation of the body temperature; myxoedematous patients complain
of feeling cold, while laboratory mammals from which the gland has
been removed (a procedure called thyroidectomy) are less resistant
to the effects of exposure to low temperature.

Whether this so-called 'calorigenic effect' of the thyroid hormones
is operative throughout the vertebrates is doubtful, for attempts to
demonstrate it in fish, either by removing the gland from dogfish or
by immobilizing it in teleosts by treating them with anti-thyroid
drugs such as thiouracil, which are known to inhibit thyroidal biosynthesis, have failed to show any convincing effect upon the oxygen
consumption of the experimental animals.   It was at one time
thought that this might be a consequence of the thyroid hormones
of lower vertebrates being different from those of mammals, but we
have seen that this cannot be so.   On the contrary, thyroxine and
tri-iodothyronine are certainly present in the thyroid glands of fish,
and it has been shown that injections of extracts of these glands will
evoke a rise in oxygen consumption when they are injected into
mammals.   We are driven to suppose, therefore, that the thyroid
hormones do not exert a calorigenic effect in the lower vertebrates,
a conclusion that is not altogether surprising, for the metabolism

of mammals is highly specialized in conjunction with the development of homoiothermy, which depends upon their possession of a basal metabolic rate much higher than that of cold-blooded forms.

Another way of looking at this problem, without wholly dismissing from consideration a possible influence of the thyroid hormones upon metabolism, is to enquire whether their action in fish may be exerted upon specific tissues rather than upon the body as a whole, so that the results of this action might not be detectable by changes in the total oxygen consumption. In this connexion it is of great interest to find that the hormones appear to play some part in the ionic exchanges involved in the osmo-regulatory processes of these animals.

A good example of this is provided by the stickleback, *Gasterosteus aculeatus*, a fish that is described as euryhaline, which means that it can withstand large changes of salinity in the external medium. Some populations of this species live for much of the year in sea-water, but when their spawning time approaches they move into fresh water, and laboratory tests with tanks that offer them a choice of different types of water show that this migration is correlated with a change in their salinity preference. During the winter they will select sea-water when given a choice between this and fresh water, but in the early spring their preference will change to a fresh-water one. The involvement of the thyroid gland in this change is shown partly by histological signs of changes in its secretory activity, but much more strikingly by the fact that fish immersed in thyroxine solution during the winter will, within a few days, develop a preference for fresh water (Fig. 36).

Among much further evidence bearing upon this problem are some observations carried out upon the starry flounder, *Platichthys stellatus*, which, like the stickleback, is also euryhaline. The interest of this evidence, which complements the above facts in an instructive way, is first, that the activity of the thyroid of the flounder, as measured by the metabolism of radioiodine, varies with the salinity of the medium in which the fish is placed, being much lower in fresh water than in sea-water. Second, and linking in a suggestive way

D 2

with the calorigenic effect, the metabolic rate of the fish is also influenced by the surrounding medium, for a marked decline in oxygen consumption is observed when animals are transferred into fresh water from the sea.

The issues involved here are not quite as simple as they may appear from this brief account, and a full consideration would necessitate correlating data obtained from the stickleback and

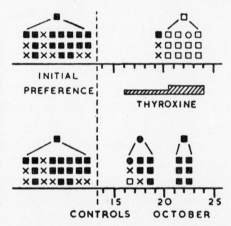

Fig. 36. Salinity preferences of stickle-backs (*Gasterosteus aculeatus*) treated with thyroxine, compared with the preferences of control animals. Open squares or circles indicate preference for fresh water; black squares or circles indicate preference for salt water; X indicates no preference. Length of horizontal bar indicates duration of phyroxine treatment, and its height indicates schematically the amount of hormone used. From Baggerman, 1959, in *Comparative Endocrinology* (A. Gorbman, ed.) (New York: Wiley).

flounder with other observations carried out upon the salmon, which is also euryhaline. Nevertheless, there is clearly some justification for the belief that the thyroid hormones may exert an influence upon the metabolism of particular cells that are involved in adaptive responses, and other considerations carry the argument further, for there is evidence that the thyroid hormones may influence cell metabolism in a more general way throughout the vertebrates.

This evidence emerges from the fact that these hormones have a growth-promoting effect in mammals, so that human infants born with defective thyroids will develop, if untreated, into cretinous dwarfs, while removal of the thyroid from young rats results in a retardation of growth. In such instances a more or less normal growth rate can be restored, both in babies and in rats, by the administration of thyroid hormones. An apparently similar effect has been demonstrated in teleost fish, for in certain species, including the rainbow trout (*Salmo gairdnerii*), immersion of young individuals in thyroxine solution may, under carefully controlled conditions, promote a marked increase in their rate of growth, both as regards length and weight (Fig. 37).

The most striking evidence for an effect of the thyroid hormones

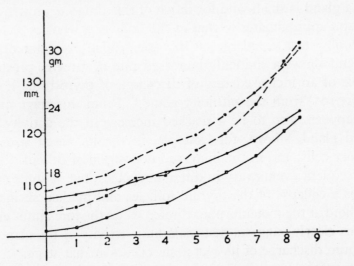

Fig. 37. Effect of thyroxine on the growth of yearling rainbow trout (*Salmo gairdnerii*). The graph shows mean weekly measurements of weight (■) and length (●) of thyroxine-treated (— — —) and control (———) groups. Abscissa, time in weeks after the beginning of the treatment. Ordinates, weight in g and length in mm. From Barrington, Piggins, and Barron, 1961, *Gen. comp. Endocrin.*, **1**, 170–178.

upon growth and development is, however, their well-known influence upon the metamorphosis of the larvae of amphibians. We have already noted that in 1912 the feeding of thyroid preparations to frog tadpoles was shown to result in premature metamorphosis, with the production of abnormally small frogs. Within a few years it had been further shown that removal of the thyroid rudiment would completely prevent them from metamorphosing, although metamorphosis could always be induced in them by the feeding of thyroid material to them. This phenomenon, which would seem the more remarkable if it were not so familiar to zoologists, has now been studied in sufficient detail to make apparent its wider implications for the analysis of thyroid function in vertebrates as a whole, and the results demonstrate particularly clearly that the closely adaptive relationship between the thyroid hormones and their target cells depends upon specialization of the latter.

During the early weeks of development of the frog tadpole its thyroid gland is small, and for much of this time the growth rate of the gland approximates to that of the body as a whole. When the hind limbs start to enlarge, at the stage called prometamorphosis, the gland shows a suddenly increased rate of growth, presumably because of an increased rate of discharge of thyrotropic hormone (pp. 31, 105) from the pituitary gland. From this stage onwards there appears also to be a marked increase in the activity of the thyroid gland, shown, for example, in the increased size of the secretory cells, and in the increased deposition of colloid. Details of subsequent events vary in different species, but in some of them there is a collapse of the thyroid follicles and marked shrinkage of the colloid at the metamorphic climax, when the fore-limbs emerge, and this clearly suggests that maximum activity of the gland, with maximum discharge of its secretion, occurs at that stage.

Fortunately our conclusions regarding the importance of the thyroid hormones in the control of these events are by no means confined to inferences drawn from the histological evidence. Studies with radioiodine have demonstrated the presence of thyroxine and of 3,5,3'-tri-iodothyronine in amphibian tadpoles, and the metabolism of this iodine has been shown to vary in a manner closely conformable with the histological appearance of the gland. Thus, in tadpoles of *Xenopus laevis* that have been treated with radioiodide the climax of metamorphosis is correlated with a marked fall in the radioiodine content of the gland, and this we may attribute to an increased rate of discharge of the hormones from it. Again, one of the indices of the hormonal content of the whole animal is the amount of protein-bound radioiodine present in it, and this also shows a significant decline in the later stages of metamorphosis, implying that there is now an increased utilization and metabolism of the hormones.

There can be no doubt, then, but that an important factor in the regulation of amphibian metamorphosis is an increasing output of thyroid hormones during the course of this process. At one time it was thought possible that the effect of this might be to produce an increased rate of metabolism in the larval tissues, but it will be obvious from what has been said earlier regarding the calorigenic effect of the thyroid hormones that this view is now outmoded. Indeed, it is a matter of dispute whether or not such an increase does actually occur and, quite apart from this, there is ample evidence that the effects of the hormones are exerted by local and direct action upon individual tissues.

This can be well demonstrated by the implantation into larvae of cholesterol pellets containing thyroxine, a device that secures slow liberation of the hormone in localized areas (cf. p. 59). It is well known that one clear-cut metamorphic event is the perforation of the operculum that makes possible the emergence of the right fore-limb. If, now, one of these pellets is inserted beneath the epidermis close to that area of the operculum in which the opening will eventually form, the rate of metamorphic change in the adjacent tissues shows a marked acceleration. The thinning and eventual perforation of the opercular wall will occur precociously, but what is of particular interest is that the neighbouring skin, which does not perforate, will show a contrasted but equally precocious response, undergoing the thickening, stratification, and cornification of its normal metamorphosis (Fig. 38). Not only, then, is the thyroxine acting locally, but superficially similar skin tissues are able to respond to it in opposite ways, a result that can only be attributed to their innate specialization.

No less striking an example of this specialization of the tissues is seen in the hind brain, where during metamorphosis two giant cells, known as Mauthner's cells, become reduced, while the neighbouring nerve cells undergo further development. These sharply contrasted responses of closely neighbouring cells can be locally evoked, just as in the case of the operculum, by the implantation of agar jelly impregnated with thyroxine.

Another aspect of this adaptation of the tissues is their sensitivity to particular concentrations of circulating thyroxine, for there is evidence that different tissues have different thresholds of response to the hormone, and these thresholds certainly vary even within one tissue according to the stage of development that it has reached.

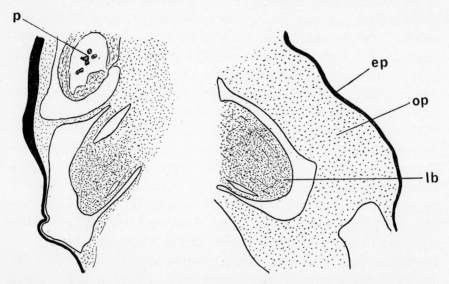

Fig. 38. Transverse sections through the opercular regions of larvae of *Rana pipiens*. *Right*, untreated control. *Left*, an experimental animal ten days after implantation of a cholesterol pellet containing thyroxine; there has been marked thinning of the opercular wall, but thickening of the epidermis above it. *ep.*, epidermis; *lb.*, fore-limb bud. *op.*, opercular wall. *p.*, encapsulated remains of pellet. Diagrammatic, from figs. 2a and 2b, Kaltenbach, 1953, *J. exp. Zool.*, **122**, 449–476.

The hind limbs are particularly sensitive, as can be shown by immersing a completely thyroidless tadpole in water containing thyroxine. If the concentration of the hormone is as low as 0·002 μg per litre, these limbs will progress from the stage with a single separate toe to the stage at which there are three separate ones, together with a common rudiment of the other two. By this stage, however, the sensitivity of the limb has declined, and an increase in concentration of thyroxine to 0·008 μg per litre will be needed to secure the further advance to a five-toed condition.

The same principle is illustrated in a rather different way by the development of the corneal reflex, which is manifested in a characteristic movement of the eyelids of amphibians when their cornea is touched. This reflex will develop in urodele tadpoles even if they are completely thyroidless and are thus incapable of metamorphosis, whereas in anuran tadpoles it develops only under the metamorphic influence of thyroxine. Thus, the two groups of amphibians clearly differ in the innate developmental capacity of homologous tissues. Moreover, implants of thyroxine-soaked agar into the hind brain of anuran tadpoles will evoke precocious development of this reflex, but only if the larva has reached an approximately mid-larval stage of development. Thyroxine is unable to accelerate this development in younger tadpoles, presumably because the tissues concerned have not yet acquired the capacity for responding to it.

It would be possible to extend this analysis further, but it must be sufficient now to add that there is some evidence that thyroxine and tri-iodothyronine differ in their capacity to induce metamorphosis. Moreover, the same is true of the analogues of these substances, for these are also capable of accelerating metamorphosis, but differ among themselves in the degree of response that they are able to evoke from different tissues. There is thus a possibility that either qualitative or quantitative variations in the secretory output of the thyroid gland, even if it be no more than variations in the relative proportions of thyroxine and tri-iodothyronine, could conceivably influence the relative degrees of response of the different tissues. As yet, however, there is no evidence to support this suggestion.

The wider implications of the hormonal regulation of amphibian metamorphosis should by now be apparent. The precise control of a diversity of reactions is seen to be mediated primarily by quantitative variations in the secretory output of the thryoid gland and by a refinement of specialization on the part of the responding cells, this specialization affecting their thresholds of response, and also the nature and the intensity of their reactions. This concept of the specialization of the target tissues is essentially what we have already postulated to explain how adaptive variations of response to the same hormones, thyroidal and steroid, are achieved at different levels of vertebrate evolution.   Obviously, then, the fact that we can observe such a mechanism at work within the body of a single individual tadpole provides a powerful reinforcement of the view that similar principles also operate in the evolution of the divergent responses of different species and groups of vertebrates.   Indeed, we may well wonder whether the evolution of hormones, as contrasted with the evolution of their effects, is a principle of any significance at all, but before we can safely attempt any decision on this issue we must consider some examples of hormones that undoubtedly do show a marked capacity for molecular variation.

4 | *Protein and Polypeptide Hormones*

Years and our trials, Mrs. Gamp, sets marks upon us all.
Charles Dickens: *Martin Chuzzlewit*

The Growth Hormone of the Pituitary Gland

THE hormones that we have so far discussed have been ones
with molecules of a comparatively simple structure, but those
with which we have now to deal are of an entirely different character, and the growth hormone of the pituitary gland is a good
example of them. The influence of this gland upon growth was
first experimentally demonstrated in 1921, when it was shown that
removal of the rudiment of the adenohypophysis of the frog tadpole at an early stage of development resulted in a reduction in
growth rate that was quite distinct from the inhibition of metamorphosis produced by removal of the thyroid gland.

This can also be readily demonstrated in the rat, for removal of
the pituitary gland (hypophysectomy) causes a decline in weight
and an arrest of skeletal growth that can be rectified by daily
implantations of adenohypophyseal tissue. Similarly, the growth of
the teleost *Fundulus heteroclitus* is arrested by hypophysectomy and
restored by injections of mammalian growth hormone. It is now
accepted, therefore, that the secretion of a growth hormone is one

of the functions of the adenohypophysis from fish up to man, and it is possible that it is also secreted in the cyclostomes, although this has not yet been established. Clearly, then, the hormonal regulation of growth is one of the fundamental features of the vertebrate endocrine system, although, as we have seen in our discussion of the thyroid hormones, the pituitary gland is not the only organ involved.

The pituitary growth hormone (often referred to simply as growth hormone, or somatotropin) is a protein, and this fact immediately reveals the difficulties involved in studying it. Hormones of low molecular weight, such as the steroids and iodo-thyronines, can be readily obtained as pure substances, either by extraction or by synthesis, and we have seen how this often makes it possible to relate differences in biological activity to differences in molecular structure. Proteins, by contrast, have very high molecular weights, and their molecules, formed by the combination of large numbers of amino acids, have a structure of extreme complexity. It is, in consequence, difficult to obtain them in a pure form; indeed, the very definition of purity becomes uncertain in this context, and the fact that a protein has been obtained in a crystalline form is no guarantee of the homogeneity of the preparation. The problems involved in determining the molecular structure of protein hormones, and the extent of their variability, are thus very complex, but there are a number of ways in which they can be attacked.

A first approximation to the characterization of the molecule is the quantitative determination of its amino-acid content and the establishment of certain constants such as the molecular weight and isoelectric point. Thus, the growth hormone of cattle has been shown to have a molecular weight of about 45,000, the molecule consisting of 393 amino-acid residues with the empirical formula:

$$\text{Glutamic acid}_{50}\text{Aspartic acid}_{35}\text{Cysteïne}_8\text{Serine}_{22}\text{Threonine}_{26}\text{-}$$
$$\text{Glycine}_{20}\text{Alanine}_{31}\text{Proline}_{14}\text{Valine}_{14}\text{Methionine}_7\text{Leucine} +$$
$$iso\text{Leucine}_{76}\text{Phenylalanine}_{27}\text{Tyrosine}_{11}\text{Lysine}_{23}\text{Histidine}_7\text{-}$$
$$\text{Arginine}_{26}\text{Tryptophan}_3(-\text{NH}_2)_{30}$$

It is also possible, given the appropriate constants, to calculate an index that expresses the shape of the molecule in terms of the axial ratio of an equivalent hydrodynamic ellipsoid, while an important relevant property is the number of cystine residues present, for these form disulphide (–S–S–) linkages that must necessarily influence that shape. Finally, an ideal end-point of all such studies, but one that is immensely difficult to reach, is the determination of the actual sequence of the amino acids in the molecule, and we shall see that even this has now been achieved for a number of the simpler polypeptide hormones.

The results of studies of pure preparations of growth hormone, obtained from teleost fish as well as from mammals, are shown in Table 2. It will be seen that they disclose a considerable range of

	Ox	Sheep	Hump-back whale	Monkey (Macacus)	Man
Molecular weight	45,000	47,400	39,900	25,400	27,100
Axial ratio of the equivalent hydrodynamic prolate ellipsoid	6·2	—	—	6·0	4·8
Isoelectric point	6·85	6·8	6·2	5·5	4·9
Number of cystine residues	4	5	3	4	2
N-terminal residue(s)	P.A	P.A	P	P	P
C-terminal sequence	A.P.P	T.A.P	L.A.P	A.G.P	T.L.P

Table 2

Some Physicochemical Properties of Various Pituitary Growth Hormones

A, alanine; *G*, glycine; *L*, leucine; *P*, phenylalanine; *T*, tyrosine. (From Geschwind, 1959, in *Comparative Endocrinology* (A. Gorbman, ed.), pp. 421–443 (New York: Wiley & Sons).

differences between the several species, and this at once raises the question whether these differences are of biological significance. Has the hormone, for example, undergone systematic evolutionary change during the history of the vertebrates, and is there any useful sense in which the higher vertebrates can be said to have retained the same growth hormone as the lower ones? Such biological problems have to be approached in biological ways, and two main techniques have been used for this purpose.

The first of these consists of administering the hormone of one species to an individual of another species, observing whether it produces a response, and determining whether such a response is greater or less than the response that the hormone normally produces in its own species. Ideally, of course, pure hormone preparations are required for such tests, and it is necessary, when pituitary hormones are under investigation, that the recipient animal should be hypophysectomized so that the results are not confused by the action of its own equivalent hormone. From the results of such biological tests it has been shown that there is, indeed, much variation in the response of particular species to growth hormones of other species. For example, the hormone of teleost fish is inactive in the rat, whereas the bovine (ox) hormone is active both in fish and in the rat. Moreover, the bovine hormone is active also in the mouse, sheep, and dog, but is inactive in the guinea-pig, rhesus monkey, and man. Again, the growth hormone of either monkey or man is active in both of these species, but is inactive in the guinea-pig and not very active in fish, while it is doubtful whether any growth hormone from species outside the Order Primates is truly active in man.

The second technique that has yielded valuable information relating to specific differences in the properties of growth hormone is the study of immunity reactions. Proteins, as well as some polysaccharides, are said to be antigens, because they are able to evoke the formation of specific antibodies when they are introduced into species other than their own. When, for example, a rabbit is given repeated injections of a protein from some other species (referred to as a heterologous species) its blood serum comes to contain an antibody capable of reacting specifically with that particular protein. The nature of this reaction will vary, but commonly the antibody is capable under suitable conditions of precipitating the antigen, in which case it is called a precipitin. These antigen–antibody reactions are part of the protective mechanism of the body, but they are also of the greatest experimental value, for their remarkably high level of specificity makes it possible to distinguish between substances that may not be distinguishable at all by ordinary chemical procedures. This principle has been developed very successfully in the analysis of the specificity of growth hormone.

The procedure adopted is to inject the hormone into a rabbit until the animal's serum contains the antibody specific to the hormone. A preparation of this serum, now referred to as anti-serum, can then be placed in a well in an agar plate and tested against hormone preparations that are placed in neighbouring wells. The

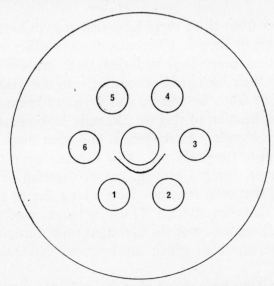

Fig. 39. Antigenic properties of growth hormones. The diagram represents an agar plate with seven wells. The centre well contains rabbit antiserum to human growth hormone. The remainder contain purified growth hormones (*1*, human; *2*, monkey; *3*, pig; *4*, whale; *5*, sheep: *6*, ox). The precipitation line that has developed between the centre well and wells *1* and *2* after 44 hours' incubation at 20–22° C indicates the close antigenic relationship between the human and monkey hormones. (Diagrammatic, after a photograph by Hayashida and Li, 1959, *Endocrinology*, **65**, 944–956).

contents of the wells diffuse through the agar, and a line of precipitation will appear if the diffusing antiserum meets a diffusing hormone with which it is able to react (Fig. 39). The occurrence of such a reaction indicates that the hormone is identical with, or closely related to, the one that was initially used to prepare the antiserum, while the absence of a reaction shows that there is no such close relationship.

The results of this procedure have shown that anti-bovine serum reacts with bovine and with ovine (sheep) hormone, but shows no reaction with the hormone of the monkey or of man. It follows that the bovine hormone must, from the immunological point of view, be closely related to the ovine, but not to those of the monkey and of man. Similarly, anti-human serum reacts with the growth hormone of the monkey or of man, but not with that of the sheep or of the ox.

It is evident from all of these facts that growth hormones from different groups or species of vertebrates show differences in their physico-chemical properties, and that these are associated with differences in their biological properties. In this respect growth hormone differs from the steroid and thyroidal hormones, and in seeking an explanation of this we naturally look first to the complexity of its molecule. Here there is one other piece of evidence that is relevant to the problem. This depends upon the fact that growth hormone, being a protein, can be digested by proteolytic enzymes, and that such enzymes show a high degree of specificity in the bonds that they attack. Thus, by selection of the enzyme, and by careful regulation of the digestion procedure, it is possible to control the extent to which the hormone molecule is broken down.

In this way it has been shown that the molecule of bovine growth hormone can be digested to an extent of 30% by chymotrypsin, and as much as 46% digested by trypsin, in both cases without any loss of its activity; evidently, then, the integrity of the original molecule is not an essential condition for the exertion of its growth-promoting effect. This has led to the suggestion that the molecule contains an 'active core', upon which its functioning depends, the remainder being removable without any impairment of that function, and this view obtains some support from the observation that the molecule of the growth hormone of man, much smaller than that of the ox, can only be 10% digested by chymotrypsin before it begins to lose its activity. We shall see later that a study of certain other hormones has provided further support for the concept of the active core, but it must be emphasized now that this concept does not necessarily imply that the remainder of the molecule is without any function at all. The means by which such a molecule exerts its effect within the body are, to say the least, obscure, but it is possible to imagine that the portion external to the core might protect the latter from degradation during its passage in the blood stream, or that it might facilitate in some way the union of that core with certain elements of the target cells that are specialized to accept it.

If, now, we attempt to set these facts within the perspective of vertebrate evolution, there is more than one way in which they can be interpreted. No doubt we must assume, as we have argued earlier, that the functioning of a hormone depends upon a close adaptive relationship between its molecules and the target cells. The fact that bovine growth hormone can influence growth in fish, but that the fish hormone is without effect in mammals, might then be explained as a result of the increased specificity of this relationship in the higher forms. The bovine hormone might retain sufficient of the primitive properties of the molecule to enable it to function in the more generalized system of fish, whereas the less specialized hormone of the latter is unable to insert itself into the more highly evolved system of mammals.

Such a situation could in theory be achieved in more than one way. The receptor system might remain unchanged, the specialization residing in the hormonal molecule, and in this case the active core might also remain unmodified, the burden of adaptive change thus resting on the remainder of the molecule. Equally, of course, the active core might itself contribute to the adaptive relationship by evolution of its own molecular structure, although the evidence from other hormones, to be considered below, indicates a strong tendency for the maintenance of stability in the core. Yet another possibility is that evolutionary specialization may modify both the receptor system of the cells and also the structure of the hormonal molecule. It is important to remember, moreover, that the tendency in evolution has been for each species of animal to develop its own characteristic complement of proteins, this, indeed, being the basis of the antigenic reactions between one species and another. Thus, the internal milieu in which a protein hormone has to function becomes modified in the course of the evolutionary history of a group, and it would seem inevitable that this in itself would make it necessary for the hormone to undergo concomitant modification if its full efficiency is to be maintained. Like Alice in Looking-Glass World, the protein components of biological systems may sometimes have to run (in an evolutionary sense) in order to remain in the same place!

Thus, there is clearly more than one possible explanation of variability in the growth hormone of vertebrates, and unfortunately we do not yet possess the information to enable us to choose between them. Nevertheless, there can be no mistaking the existence here of a variability differing in extent and character from any that we have encountered in the simpler steroid and thyroidal molecules, nor is this variability confined to the growth hormone alone. Other hormones are also secreted by the adeno-hypophysis, and sufficient is now known of some of these to indicate that the above considerations are equally applicable to them.

The Gonadotropic and Thyrotropic Hormones of the Pituitary Gland

Two examples of these hormones are provided by follicle-stimulating hormone (FSH) and interstitial-cell-stimulating hormone (ICSH, also known as luteinizing hormone, or LH). We have already noted that these are called gonadotropic hormones because they exert a regulatory influence upon the gonads. It will be sufficient now to add that FSH takes its name from the stimulatory influence that it exerts upon the development of the Graafian follicles of the mammalian ovary, while ICSH stimulates the development of the steroid-secreting interstitial tissue of the testes, and probably of the corresponding tissue in the ovaries. These two hormones are complex proteins, which, unlike the protein of growth hormone, are conjugated with a carbohydrate component, in which respect they resemble thyroglobulin. They are termed either glycoproteins or mucoproteins, according to whether the amount of the carbohydrate hexosamine that they contain is respectively less or more than 4%.

These two hormones, like growth hormone, have antigenic properties, and purified preparations from sheep pituitaries have been used to prepare rabbit antisera against each of them. Tests carried out like those described above show, as might be expected, that a precipitin reaction develops between ovine FSH antiserum and ovine FSH. Particularly interesting, however, in the light of our previous discussion is the fact that no reaction occurs when ovine FSH antiserum is tested against various heterologous preparations that are known to contain FSH activity, including extracts of the pituitary of rats, of the serum of pregnant mares, and of the urine either of pregnant women or of those who have passed the menopause. This indicates that hormonal molecules can be immunologically distinct from each other, even though they possess a similar type of biological activity. Now FSH activity is known not to be species specific, for a gonadotropic effect can be induced in one species by a FSH from another species, and it follows that we have here some supporting evidence for the view that the antigenic property of the FSH molecules lies in a region separate from the hormonally active core.

One further example is provided by thyrotropin, the glycoprotein hormone of the adenohypophysis that is responsible for the regulation of the activity of the thyroid gland. This hormone is present throughout the vertebrates, from fish to man, and perhaps also in the Cyclostomata, and it has thus been possible to obtain preparations of it from various groups of vertebrates, and to study their influence upon the activity of the thyroid gland as expressed in its rate of uptake of radioiodide.

In this way it has been shown that pituitary extracts from various species of teleosts will produce a marked increase in the activity of the thyroid gland when they are injected into eels that have been deprived of their own thyrotropin by previous hypophysectomy. Similar positive responses are obtained from rainbow trout in which thyroid activity has been depressed by starvation. These results are the expected ones, and they demonstrate the presence of thyrotropin in the extracts. If, however, identical extracts are injected into mice no significant response is evoked, a negative result that recalls the comparable one obtained when mammals are treated with the growth hormone of fish.

One possible explanation of these results would be that the fish pituitary extracts contained some substance inhibitory to the action of the thyroid gland of mammals, but investigation of this possibility has given no evidence in favour of it. An alternative explanation is that the thyrotropin molecule has undergone evolutionary change during the history of the vertebrates, and that this has resulted, as we have suggested for growth hormone, in an increasingly close adaptive relationship between the hormone and its target cells in the thyroid gland. This would explain, theoretically, why the mammalian hormone can influence the thyroid of fish, and why the fish hormone cannot influence the more specialized system of the mammal.

If this argument is well founded it might be expected that pituitaries of vertebrates at an intermediate stage of evolution might well be able to stimulate the mammalian thyroid, and this has, in fact, been found to be so, for the injection into rats of extracts of the pituitary of frogs does increase the uptake of radioiodine into the thyroid gland. This suggests that the results of such experiments depend upon the phylogenetic status of the animals concerned, and further evidence for this has been obtained by preparing pituitary extracts from the lung-fish, *Protopterus*. The significance of this animal is that the lung-fish are of all living fish (with the exception, perhaps, of the coelacanth *Latimeria*), the closest to the tetrapod vertebrates, while it is known that the pituitary gland of *Protopterus* is remarkably like that of amphibians in its organization. It is thus of interest that these extracts differ from those of teleost fish, and resemble those of frogs, in activating the thyroid gland of mammals. Ideally, of course, these results need to be confirmed with pure preparations of thyrotropin from the species concerned, but even in the absence of these there still remains a suggestion that the biochemical evolution of the hormone may be running parallel to the morphological evolution of the pituitary gland by which it is secreted.

One other aspect of these studies of thyrotropin merits attention, and this is the influence of temperature upon the activity of the hormone. When mammalian extracts are tested upon fish at two different temperatures, 20° and 10° C, their activity at the lower temperature is markedly less than at the higher one. When, however, fish extracts are tested upon fish in the same way there is no appreciable difference in the activity of the extracts at the two temperatures. This is another indication of a difference between the properties of the thyrotropin of fish and of mammals, and it is possible to argue that it might be an adaptive one, for the mammalian hormone has always to act at the constant high temperature of the mammalian body, whereas the hormone of fish, operating within the body of a poikilotherm, has to function over a wider temperature range.

Whether this is the correct interpretation is, however, by no means clear, for in this respect also the hormone of *Protopterus* resembles that of mammals rather than that of fish, since it shows a marked decline in its activity at the lower temperature. This can hardly be adaptive in the sense just outlined, and must presumably be attributed to some similarity of structure between the hormone of the lung-fish and that of mammals. If this be so, it would seem to follow that the supposedly adaptive thermal sensitivity of the mammalian hormone was achieved in advance of the development of homoiothermy, which would place it within the category of what are called pre-adaptations. These are properties that appear in advance of any biological need for them, but which by their existence facilitate later evolutionary developments, and we have already seen one possible illustration of them in the fact that progesterone existed before the establishment of the mammalian reproductive mechanism. However, it is probably wiser to regard the information available at this stage as being too fragmentary to allow us to judge whether such an interpretation is also applicable to the history of thyrotropin.

It will be apparent that we have now been led in our argument not only to the recognition of variability in the molecules of protein hormones, associated with a considerable measure of species and group specificity, but also to a suggestion that in some circumstances such variability might have been turned to adaptive advantage during the course of vertebrate history. We have, however, been limited in our conclusions by ignorance of the precise structure of the molecules concerned, and by the consequent impossibility of linking molecular variation with biological activity in the manner that proved so instructive when we were considering steroid and thyroidal hormones. It is fortunate, therefore, that these arguments can be tested further by considering certain other hormonal molecules that are properly described as polypeptides. These, like the protein hormones, show a clearly-defined molecular variation, but their molecular structure is simpler, and this has made it possible to determine the precise arrangement of the amino acids of which they are composed.

Molecular Variation in Polypeptide Hormones

Most of the polypeptide hormones with which we are concerned are associated with the pituitary, but one that is not, and that merits prior mention, is insulin, for it was the studies of Sanger on the molecular structure of this hormone that facilitated the subsequent analysis of the others.

Insulin, secreted, as we have seen, by the islets of Langerhans of the pancreas, has far-reaching effects upon metabolism, and it is well known that in its absence there is a profound disturbance of carbohydrate relationships within the body, resulting in the wasting condition known as diabetes mellitus, in which glucose is passed in the urine and lost to the organism. Owing to its immense clinical importance, the problem of the structure of the insulin molecule has attracted much attention ever since the discovery of the hormone in 1921, and already by the 1940s it was known to be composed of relatively short polypeptide chains. This fact, together with estimates of the molecular weight (now known to be about 6,000), indicated that the molecule was very much smaller than those that we have just discussed, and that there was thus some prospect of being able to determine its precise structure. A variety of micro-chemical procedures were used for this, the underlying principle being to disrupt the molecule (by partial hydrolysis, for example) and then to determine the amino-acid components of the fragments.

The complete structure of the molecule of bovine insulin, as

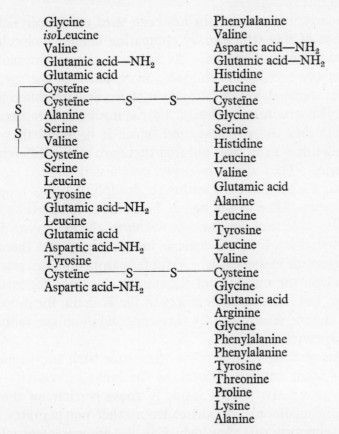

Glycine   Phenylalanine
*iso*Leucine   Valine
Valine   Aspartic acid—NH$_2$
Glutamic acid—NH$_2$ Glutamic acid—NH$_2$
Glutamic acid   Histidine
Cysteïne   Leucine
Cysteïne——————S——————S——————Cysteïne
Alanine   Glycine
Serine   Serine
Valine   Histidine
Cysteïne   Leucine
Serine   Valine
Leucine   Glutamic acid
Tyrosine   Alanine
Glutamic acid–NH$_2$ Leucine
Leucine   Tyrosine
Glutamic acid   Leucine
Aspartic acid–NH$_2$ Valine
Tyrosine   Cysteine
Cysteïne——————S——————S——————Cysteine
Aspartic acid–NH$_2$ Glycine
                                           Glutamic acid
                                           Arginine
                                           Glycine
                                           Phenylalanine
                                           Phenylalanine
                                           Tyrosine
                                           Threonine
                                           Proline
                                           Lysine
                                           Alanine

Fig. 40. Amino-acid sequences of the insulin molecule of the ox; the A-chain is to the left and the B-chain to the right. After Sanger, 1960, *Brit. med. Bull.* **16**, 183–188, from Barrington, 1962, *Introduction to General and Comparative Endocrinology* (Oxford: Clarendon Press).

revealed by these methods, is shown in Fig. 40, from which it will be seen that it consists of two polypeptide chains, the longer (B) chain containing 30 amino-acid residues while the shorter (A) chain contains 21. The two are joined by disulphide bridges, and this feature is essential for the activity of the molecule, which is immediately inactivated if they are broken either by reduction or by oxidation. Another disulphide bridge is present as part of the A chain, but there is no evidence that this is of the same functional importance as the others.

Particularly interesting light has been shed on the physiological significance of this structure by comparing insulin molecules obtained from different species. As far as is known, the biological activity of the hormone is the same irrespective of the species in which it is secreted, yet despite this it shows specific differences in its molecular structure. Thus, if bovine insulin is compared with that of the pig, sheep, horse, and whale it is found that the B chain is identical in all five, but that there are minor differences in the A chain. They affect, however, only a very limited length of that chain, the portion lying within its disulphide bridge; here the alanine–serine–valine of the bovine hormone is replaced by threonine–serine–*iso*leucine in the pig, alanine–glycine–valine in the sheep, threonine–glycine–*iso*leucine in the horse, and threonine–serine–*iso*leucine in the whale. As for human insulin, this resembles in its A chain the molecule of the pig, as also does the insulin of the rabbit, but there are differences in the B chain, for in man the terminal alanine is replaced by threonine, while in the rabbit it is replaced by serine.

It seems reasonable to suppose that since such substitutions as these can occur without influencing the biological activity of the molecule, that activity must reside in those portions of the chain that remain unaltered. Evidence from other polypeptides, as we shall see, supports this view, which is also in agreement with the belief that the activity of protein hormones depends upon an active core in their molecules, although the structural situation in them is naturally much more complex. From the evolutionary point of view we must necessarily ask why such substitutions should occur at all, and our discussion of growth hormone has shown that there is no simple answer to this question. Current views assume that the arrangement of amino acids in the proteins secreted by the cell is primarily determined by the nuclear deoxyribonucleic acid

(DNA), which is conceived as fulfilling the role of a template. If this is so, it may well be that any one amino-acid substitution is the consequence of a single gene mutation, so that our question really resolves itself into the problem of how such a mutation comes to be established in the first instance.

If we assume that this must depend upon the action of natural selection we may reasonably look for the mutation to have some positive survival value, for without this, according to the mathematical analysis of the action of natural selection, no mutation can be expected to spread through a species. No doubt it is possible that such slight changes may improve the adaptive relationship between the hormone and its target cells in the unique internal environment that we have seen is provided by each individual species, but it is also possible that they are of no immediate value at all. The pleiotropic effects of genes, to which we have earlier referred, may very well result in a particular mutation having irrelevant and unimportant side influences, while its primary action, the one for which it is selected, may be exerted in quite another direction. On the other hand, it is certain that such side influences provide a reserve of variability upon which a species can draw should new adaptational needs create new selection pressure, and to this extent the variability of polypeptide and protein hormones constitutes theoretically a measure of pre-adaptation to changing circumstances. We know too little of the range of variability in the insulin molecule to take this argument very far, but if we now pass to consider other polypeptide hormones we shall see that they give it some support.

Corticotropin, the pituitary hormone that regulates the activity of the adrenocortical tissue, is known to be a straight-chain polypeptide containing 39 amino-acid residues (Fig. 41). This hormone has been isolated from pituitaries of the ox, sheep, pig, and man, and comparative studies have revealed specific differences of the same character as those just discussed. This is apparent even from the results of amino-acid analysis, which shows that the bovine, ovine, and human hormones are of identical composition, but that the pig hormone differs in containing two residues of

serine and two of leucine, whereas the others contain three of serine
and one of leucine.

The establishment of the complete molecular structure of the
corticotropins of the ox, sheep, and pig has shown that these
substitutions occur in positions 31 and 32, the serine–alanine of
the ox becoming leucine–alanine in the pig.   In addition, there are
further differences that are not apparent in the total amino-acid

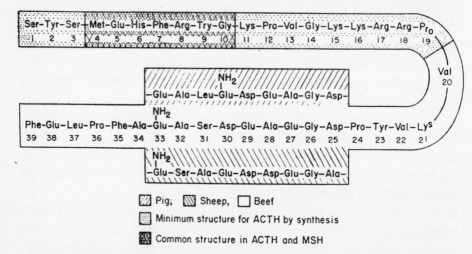

Fig. 41.   Structure of the corticotropin (ACTH) molecule.   For a guide to the
amino acids, here and in Fig. 42, refer to Fig. 40.   From Li, 1962, *Gen. comp.
Endocrin., Supplement 1,* 8–11.

analysis, for these same serine–alanine residues of the ox are reversed to alanine–serine in the sheep, and other differences in
sequence are found in positions 25 to 29.   These, then, appear to
be true specific variations, as far as we can judge from this limited
information, and are fully comparable with those of insulin.

According to our earlier argument, we should expect to find
that the biological activity of the corticotropin molecule resides
within the region that is not affected by these substitutions, for
there is no evidence that they affect its activity in any way at all.
Strong evidence in support of that argument comes from studies of
the activities of fragments released by partial hydrolysis of the
molecule, for these have shown that a portion consisting of the

first 24 positions retains full activity, and that this is the smallest portion that does do so. On this evidence, then, the amino-acid substitutions and rearrangements so far reported all occur within a length of the molecule that is not essential for securing its full activity.

A final and completely convincing demonstration of the structural requirements for full corticotropic activity really demands the synthesis of a polypeptide chain that can then be shown to be the minimal requirement for matching the activity of the intact molecule, and much progress towards this point has been achieved with the synthesis of a nonadecapeptide that contains positions 1 to 19, and that has been found to carry about 50% of the complete activity.

The importance of these structural studies of the corticotropin molecule extends much further, however, than we have so far indicated, for the hormone has long been known to be associated in some way with the responses of the pigment-containing cells (chromatophores) of the lower vertebrates. The capacity of many of these animals to change colour in response to various stimuli, including the colour of their background and the intensity of the illumination to which they are exposed, depends in part upon the effecting of a long-term increase or reduction of the total amount of pigment in their skin, a phenomenon known as morphological colour change. In addition, there are the more rapid responses that result from the dispersal or concentration of the pigment granules within the chromatophores; these constitute the phenomenon known as physiological colour change, and it is well established that they are regulated by the pituitary gland, as also, perhaps, is the morphological type of response.

In elasmobranchs and amphibians the regulation is probably entirely hormonal, while in teleosts and reptiles it is partly hormonal and partly mediated by the direct action of the autonomic nervous system upon the cells. The hormone mainly (and perhaps exclusively) concerned is secreted by the pars intermedia of the adenohypophysis, and for that reason it has commonly been called intermedin, although it is now becoming more usual to call it melanocyte-stimulating hormone (MSH). This term arises from the fact that it has been investigated almost exclusively with reference to its effect upon the melanocytes (or melanophores), those chromatophores that contain the dark melanin pigments.

MSH occurs throughout the vertebrates, and not only in those lower forms that show physiological colour change, and this circumstance has made it possible to extract it from mammalian pituitaries in quantities sufficient to enable its molecular structure to be established. Particular attention has been given to these studies because corticotropin preparations have long been known to have some melanocyte-stimulating activity, a fact that, together with certain clinical observations, led at one time to the suggestion that the two hormones might actually be identical. It is now known that this is not so, but the facts revealed are nevertheless of the greatest interest.

A fundamental conclusion from the structural investigations is that MSH is a hormone complex, a situation that has now been so widely demonstrated for so many hormones (adrenaline and nor-adrenaline, for example, and thyroxine and 3,5,3′-tri-iodothyro-nine) that it almost appears to be a basic principle of endocrine organization. Two primary hormones have been isolated and characterized (Fig. 42), and these are known respectively as α-MSH and β-MSH, the former having a higher isoelectric point. α-MSH, the more basic of the two, is a polypeptide composed of 13 amino-acid residues, one end of the chain having an N-acetyl-serine and the other a valine amide, and this structure, which has been confirmed by complete synthesis of the molecule, has been shown to occur also in the hormone of the ox, pig, and horse.

The structure of β-MSH has been determined for the same three species, and has been shown to be a chain of 18 amino-acid residues, but in this instance with some specific differences. As may be seen from Fig. 42, the bovine hormone differs from that of the pig in that serine is substituted for glutamic acid at position 2. In this respect the hormone of the horse resembles that of the pig, but it nevertheless differs from the hormones both of that animal and of the ox in having arginine substituted for proline at position

ACTH: (Pig, Sheep, Beef)
Ser.1 Tyr.2 Ser.3 | Met.4 Glu.5 His.6 Phe.7 Arg.8 Try.9 Gly.10 Lys.11 Pro.12 | Val.13 Gly.14 Lys.15 Lys.16 Arg.17 Arg.18 Pro.19

α-MSH: (Pig, Beef, Horse)
CH₃CO Ser.1 Tyr.2 Ser.3 Met.4 Glu.5 His.6 Phe.7 Arg.8 Try.9 Gly.10 Lys.11 Pro.12 Val.13 NH₂

β-MSH: (Pig)
Asp.1 Glu.2 Gly.3 Pro.4 | Tyr.5 Lys.6 Met.7 Glu.8 His.9 Phe.10 Arg.11 Try.12 Gly.13 Ser.14 Pro.15 | Pro.16 Lys.17 Asp.18

β-MSH: (Beef)
Asp.1 Ser.2 Gly.3 Pro.4 Tyr.5 Lys.6 Met.7 Glu.8 His.9 Phe.10 Arg.11 Try.12 Gly.13 Ser.14 Pro.15 Pro.16 Lys.17 Asp.18

β-MSH: (Horse)
Asp.1 Glu.2 Gly.3 Pro.4 Tyr.5 Lys.6 Met.7 Glu.8 His.9 Phe.10 Arg.11 Try.12 Gly.13 Ser.14 Pro.15 Arg.16 Lys.17 Asp.18

β-MSH: (Human)
Ala.1 Glu.2 Lys.3 Lys.4 Asp.5 Glu.6 Gly.7 Pro.8 | Tyr.9 Arg.10 Met.11 Glu.12 His.13 Phe.14 Arg.15 Try.16 Gly.17 Ser.18 Pro.19 | Pro.20 Lys.21 Asp.22

Fig. 42. The relationships between the structure of the molecules of the melanocyte-stimulating hormones and of part of the molecule of corticotropin (ACTH). From Li, 1961, *Vitamins and Hormones*, **19**, 313–329.

16. Finally, the β-MSH of man differs from all three in the presence of additional amino acids at one end.

Now if the structural formulae of the melanocyte-stimulating hormones are compared with that of corticotropin the interesting fact emerges that all of them, including corticotropin itself, possess a common heptapeptide sequence, representing positions 4 to 10 of corticotropin and of α-MSH, and 7 to 13 of the β-MSH of the pig, ox, and horse (Figs. 41, 42). This immediately suggests that this particular sequence may be responsible for melanocyte-stimulating activity, and some confirmation of this has been secured by the study of a variety of synthetic peptides, which has shown that the shortest amino-acid chain to possess this activity is a pentapeptide representing positions 6 to 10 of corticotropin. It does not, however, show anything approaching the full activity of the intact molecules, and study of other synthetic products makes it clear that melanocyte-stimulating capacity increases as the chain is extended from either end.

Further comparison of the formulae (Fig. 42) shows that the resemblance between corticotropin and the melanocyte-stimulating hormones goes still further, for the α-MSH chain is identical with positions 1 to 13 of corticotropin, apart from the acetyl group at one end and the amide group at the other. Then again, the complete array of melanocyte-stimulating hormones shows a sequence of 11 amino-acid residues which differs from the sequence of positions 2 to 12 of the corticotropin chain in no more than the interchange of serine and lysine at two positions.

Such close correspondence, combined with overlapping of biological activity, cannot be a coincidence; indeed, we shall see an analogous example when we consider the polypeptide hormones of the hypothalamus and neurohypophysis. In the present instance it seems relevant that the pars distalis, secreting corticotropin, and the pars intermedia, secreting the melanocyte-stimulating hormones, are differentiated out of a common embryonic forerunner, the adenohypophysis (p. 28), for this suggests that this particular group of hormones may have arisen by the evolutionary modification of a common ancestral molecule, or biosynthetic pattern, that was a property of the adenohypophysis at a very early stage of its history. We should appear, in fact, to have here another possible example of adaptive radiation at the molecular level, analogous to that mentioned earlier in our discussion of the steroid hormones.

Physiological colour change, apparently dependent upon MSH, is already established in the cyclostomes, but it is still uncertain whether or not corticotropin is present in them. We cannot, therefore, plot the possible course of this molecular evolution in any detail, but we can feel sure that it must have been initiated at an early stage of vertebrate history, for there is some evidence that the adrenocortical tissue of fish is certainly under pituitary control. The significance of the diversification of the melanocyte-stimulating hormones is obscure, although the same considerations apply here as in the case of the specific variation of growth hormone and of corticotropin, and need not be repeated. There is certainly no reason to believe that it is purely a mammalian phenomenon, for chromatographic studies have already indicated the presence of more than one type of MSH molecule in fish and in amphibians, and it seems possible that the variants are not always identical with those isolated from mammals.

It is of interest that when β-MSH is injected into hypophys-ectomized frogs the hormones of the pig and horse are as much as five times more effective than is that of the ox in evoking pigment dispersal. Evidently, then, the substitution at position 2 must have some influence upon melanocyte-stimulating activity, while the extension of the chain at the other end must have been the main factor involved in the establishment of corticotropic activity. It would appear, therefore, that the polypeptide chain is a type of molecular structure that lends itself well to the provision of a reserve of variation, or at least to a potentiality for establishing this. Such a reserve, as we have already suggested, could, in theory, be a valuable factor in facilitating the continued adaptive evolution of a group, for it constitutes a store of variation upon which natural selection can draw as new needs arise. The degree to which animal groups have actually made use of this potentiality, however, and the extent to which it makes unnecessary the evolution of adaptive modification in the target cells of such hormones, are questions that we shall be able better to consider when we deal with the hormones of the hypothalamus and neurohypophysis.

It remains to comment on the puzzling fact that the melanocyte-stimulating hormones persist in birds and mammals, for these animals no longer possess the capacity for physiological colour change. One suggested explanation is that the hormones are biochemical vestiges, lacking any function, and explicable only in terms of past evolutionary history, but it would be unwise to adopt this view until much more attention has been given to the possibility that they may still possess some function that is of significance in the life of higher vertebrates.

There is, in fact, evidence that injection of these hormones into human beings can darken the colour of the skin, which suggests that they may still be involved in some way with the metabolism of the skin pigments. It is also possible that they may have acquired new functions, or that they possess functions in the lower vertebrates that have not yet been discovered, and that are still manifested in birds and mammals. These are matters that are attracting attention at the present time, but no decisive conclusions have yet emerged, and the problem remains one of the many that have still to be unravelled by comparative endocrinological research.

Hormones and Colour Change in Invertebrates

Far too little is known of the nature of invertebrate hormones to permit of any discussion comparable in detail with the above. Nevertheless, it is relevant to recall at this point that physiological colour change is found in many groups of these animals, including the crustaceans and certain insects. It is particularly prominent in the higher Crustacea, which possess chromatophores that are similar in general character to those of the vertebrates, and resemble the latter also in being regulated by hormones. There is a difference in this respect, however, in that the MSH of vertebrates is secreted by glandular tissue of the adenohypophysis, whereas the chromactivating hormones of crustaceans are neurosecretory products.

In contrast to this, the physiological colour change of the stick insect *Carausius* (*Dixippus*) depends upon chromatophores that are of a peculiar type, being simply a part of the surface epithelium, yet its controlling system resembles the crustacean one in that it comprises neurosecretory hormones associated with the brain and corpora cardiaca, which, as we have seen, correspond closely with the X organ and sinus gland of crustaceans. In this instance, then, we have a similar pattern of endocrine organization in two closely related groups, and it is the more unfortunate that as yet we know nothing of the molecular structure of the hormones concerned, although the use of electrophoresis has at least made it possible to compare some of the properties of active and highly purified extracts of the relevant neurosecretory centres.

This has shown that a so-called A-substance, capable of concentrating the pigment granules in the large and the small red chromatophores of the prawn *Palaemon*, can be extracted from the sinus gland and post-commissure organs of that animal, and that a substance with identical properties is also extractable from the corpora cardiaca of *Carausius*. Subject to the necessary reservation that identical biological effects may be produced by molecules of different structure (p. 57), this certainly suggests that there may be some degree of chemical identity in the products of the neurosecretory centres concerned. Since these centres are themselves so similar in their anatomical organization, there is here another interesting hint of correspondence between the molecular and morphological levels of analysis (p. 116). Much more information is needed, however, before this correspondence can be argued with any degree of assurance.

Certainly there are differences between these secretions, for *Palaemon* extracts contain a B-substance, concentrating the red pigment in the large chromatophores and dispersing that in the small ones, but this is not found in *Carausius*. Conversely, the latter secretes a C-substance that is not found in crustacean extracts, and that has no effect on the chromatophores of *Palaemon*, although it concentrates the dark pigment in the shrimp *Crangon*.

Finally, it would be natural to enquire whether any of these chromactivating substances bear any relationship at all to the melanocyte-stimulating molecules of vertebrates. There is, in fact, some evidence in earlier work that pituitary extracts of vertebrates can evoke responses in crutacean chromatophores, but this needs re-examination, for in the light of more recent developments in this field it is of rather doubtful significance. Having regard to our earlier discussion of the implications of phylogenetic relationships (p. 39), we might well expect to find that the molecular patterns of invertebrate chromactivating hormones are different from those of vertebrates; it is well, however, to be prepared to find nature surprising us with wholly unexpected situations.

5 The Polypeptide Hormones of the Hypothalamus

This is all very well, Mr. Nickleby, and very proper, so far as it goes—
so far as it goes, but it doesn't go far enough.
Charles Dickens: *Nicholas Nickleby*

Oxytocin and Vasopressin

THE first demonstration of the biological activity of the neuro-hypophysis followed closely on the discovery of the vasopressor action of extracts of the adrenal gland, for it was soon found that a similar result was obtained when extracts of the posterior lobes of the pituitary glands of cattle were injected into mammals. Later it became apparent that this activity was actually located in the neural lobe, and in the course of time it was found that other biological activities, to be mentioned below, were also detectable in that region. It is not clear, even at the present day, whether or not all of these activities are truly hormonal in nature, but two of them certainly are, and they are now known to be properties of two distinct hormones, oxytocin and vasopressin.

We have seen that the neural lobe is not a true endocrine gland, but a neurohaemal release centre, which means that these two hormones are not produced in the neural lobe but are passed into it along the axons of neurosecretory cells located in the hypothalamus. They are thus properly to be regarded as hypothalamic hormones, and confirmatory evidence for this is to be seen in their distribution, for they are demonstrable in extracts of the hypothalamus, as well as in extracts of the neural lobe itself.   Moreover, certain conditions that result in the discharge of one or other of the hormones into the blood stream produce a reduction of neurosecretory material not only in the neural lobe but also in the neurosecretory centres and axons of the hypothalamus.   This does not mean that the neuro-secretory substance that is visible in suitably stained sections of these regions consists merely of the hormones.   On the contrary, it is generally believed that these are secreted and transmitted in loose combination with protein, and that it is the latter that is actually visible.   As for the hormones, there is now completely convincing evidence that they are simple polypeptides, and the study of these, and of closely related compounds that have been synthesized in the laboratory, has produced results that are of the greatest evolutionary interest.

In order to appreciate these it is necessary to understand that there are two main types of procedure by which these polypeptides can be identified and characterized.   The first, which involves the chemical determination of their amino-acid content, and the establishment of the arrangement of the amino-acid residues within their molecules, may be said to have been initiated in 1933 with the isolation and purification of oxytocin, and with the determination of its complete molecular structure.   Oxytocin has been identified in neurohypophyseal extracts of cattle, pigs, sheep, horses, and humans, and in each of these species its molecular structure has been checked by amino-acid analysis and has been shown to be always the same (Fig. 43).   It may be thought of as comprising a straight chain of 8 amino-acids; one of these, however, is cystine, with its disulphide ($-S-S-$) linkage, so that in fact the molecule is formed of a ring, which includes the two half-cystine (cysteïne) residues, and a side chain.   It is thus customary to identify the amino-acid residues by numbering them from 1 to 9, starting with the terminal cysteïne.

By 1955 the molecular structure of the vasopressin of the ox had also been determined (Fig. 43), and had been shown to correspond very closely with that of oxytocin.   In this form, known as arginine

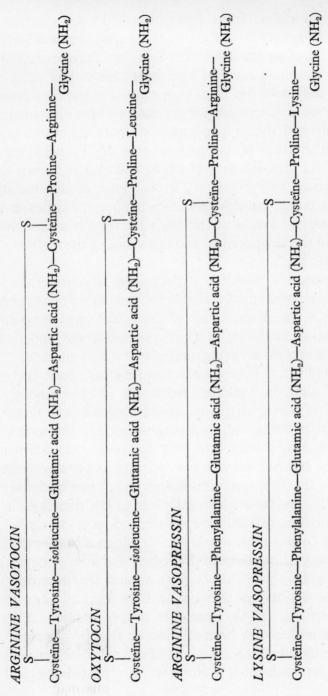

Fig. 43. Amino-acid sequences of the molecules of the hypothalamic polypeptide hormones.

E

vasopressin, it differs from oxytocin only in the substitution of phenylalanine for *iso*leucine at position 3, and arginine for leucine at position 8. An identical hormone has been extracted from neurohypophyseal extracts of the sheep, horse, and man, but an interesting difference has been encountered in the Suiformes. In this group the peccary secretes arginine vasopressin, whereas the domestic pig and the hippopotamus do not; all three, however, secrete another form of vasopressin, that differs in having lysine substituted for arginine at position 8, and that is known for this reason as lysine vasopressin. The existence of this variation in molecular structure immediately raises the question whether similar variations might have been the basis for the divergence between oxytocin and the vasopressins, and this is one of the matters that we shall examine later.

Before doing this, however, it is necessary to consider the second of the two types of method available for identifying these hormones. This involves the determining of their biological properties by pharmacological methods, in which the substances under test are either administered to living animals (*in vivo* methods) or are applied to individual organs or tissues that have been excised and maintained alive in suitable media (*in vitro* methods). The description of these methods as pharmacological rather than physiological is deliberate, and means that the properties under investigation do not necessarily play any part in the normal functioning of the animal from which the substances have been extracted, a reservation that in no wise diminishes their value as characteristic properties that can be used for purposes of identification.

Indeed, what makes this group of methods particularly helpful is that there is considerable overlap in the distribution of properties among the several hormones. Biological activities of oxytocin, for example, are also shown, although to a much less intensity, by the vasopressins, a situation that no doubt reflects the fact that the molecular structure of the hormones is very similar. A series of such properties has now been studied, so that by determining the activity of each substance in respect of each of these properties it is possible to establish for it a characteristic 'pharmacological spectrum', which can then be compared, item by item, with corresponding 'spectra' determined for other substances (Table 3). In this way differences can be defined, and identifications confirmed, with an assurance that would be impossible if reliance had to be placed upon only one or two such properties. It also becomes practicable to attempt to relate each of these properties to particular features of molecular structure, thereby extending the type of analysis that we

Assay method	Arginine vasotocin	Arginine vasopressin	Lysine vasopressin	Oxytocin
Rat uterus	40	20–25	15–20	360, 415
Rat blood pressure	71	400–450	270–340	<10, 3·8
Rat antidiuresis	71	400–450	110–140	diuretic
Rabbit milk ejection	119	70–80	50–60	371
Hen oviduct	1630	320	29	29
Frog water balance	2600	—	—	(360)
Frog bladder	7800	21	<5	360

Table 3

Comparison of the Potency of Hypothalamic Neuropophyseal Hormones (Expressed as Milliunits per μg), Assayed against the Third International Standard Powder

Data collected from various sources by Heller and Pickering, 1961, *J. Physiol.*, **155**, 98–114.

have already encountered in considering certain other polypeptide hormones.

It is not possible here to do more than refer very briefly to the various components of these spectra, but they can be summarized under the following main headings:

1. *Rat Vasopressor Activity*, indicated by the rise in blood pressure produced by intravenous injection into rats (Fig. 44). This activity, which is particularly characteristic of vasopressin, is markedly dependent upon the presence at position 8 of the highly basic amino-acid arginine; it is progressively diminished, therefore, by substituting lysine, histidine, or leucine for arginine, so that lysine vasopressin is less active in this regard than is arginine vasopressin. Whether this vasopressor activity is of any physiological significance in normal animals remains very doubtful, and it may be no more than a pharmacological property of the molecule.

2. *Rat Antidiuresis Activity*, indicated by a reduction or inhibition of the flow of urine in rats following intravenous injection.

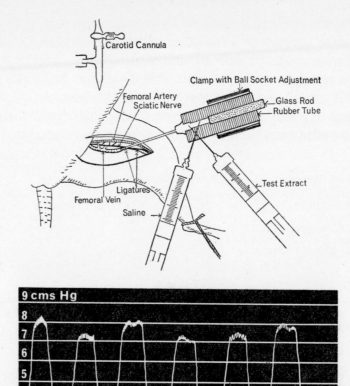

Fig. 44. *Above*, apparatus used for recording the vasopressor action of the hypothalamic polypeptide hormones. Preparations are injected into the femoral
vein, and the blood pressure recorded through a cannula inserted into the
carotid artery. *Below*, tracing showing the results obtained by this method.
Abscissae, time; ordinates, blood pressure. The injections were: *25*, 0·008
international units of a posterior lobe extract; *26*, 0·006; *27*, 0·008; *28*, 0·006;
29, 0·006; *30*, 0·008; *Sa.*, 0·2 ml saline. From Landgrebe *et al.*, 1946, *Proc.
Roy. Soc. Edin.* **B 62**, 202–210.

This, too, is particularly characteristic of vasopressin, and probably
results from the hormone modifying the permeability of certain
parts of the kidney tubules. Unlike the vasopressor activity of
vasopressin, this is unquestionably a true hormonal effect, of great
importance in the regulation of water balance in mammals. Its

influence is dramatically shown in man, where a lack of this hormone leads to the condition of diabetes insipidus, in which an excessive output of urine may necessitate the drinking of as much as 30 litres of water per day.

3. *Rat Uterus Activity*, indicated by the evoking of contractions of the uterus either *in vivo* or *in vitro*. This activity is particularly characteristic of oxytocin, and constitutes the 'oxytocic' effect from which that hormone takes its name. It might well be supposed

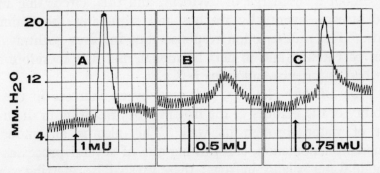

Fig. 45. The effect of intravenous injections of standard pituitary extract on the pressure in the lactating mammary gland of a lactating rabbit; the animal weighed 1·8 kg, and was in the eighth day of lactation. The small regular waves represent respiratory movements. One division on the abscissa represents 2 sec. After Thorp, 1962, in *Methods in Hormone Research* (R. I. Dorfman, ed.), **2**, 495–516 (New York: Academic Press).

that it would be of physiological importance, particularly at parturition, but it is far from certain that this is actually so; like the vasopressor effect, this may be only a pharmacological property of the molecule.

4. *Hen Oviduct Activity*, indicated *in vitro* by the evoking of contractions in strips from the wall of the oviduct of the fowl.

5. *Fowl Vasodepressor Activity*, indicated by a fall in arterial pressure in the chick after injection.

6. *Rabbit Milk-ejection Activity*, indicated by a rise in pressure in the mammary ducts after injection into lactating rabbits (Fig. 45). This is particularly characteristic of oxytocin, and, like the antidiuretic activity of vasopressin, is an undoubted hormonal property, and one that constitutes an essential element in the complex process

of lactation. During this process the milk collects in the alveoli and finer ducts of the mammary glands, and is expelled from them by contraction of the smooth muscle of their walls. This contraction takes place in response to stimulation of the teat, either by the suckling of the young or, in domestic stock, by the hands of the milker. The stimulation results in the transmission of nerve impulses from the sensory elements of the teats into the brain; here they are directed into the hypothalamus and neural lobe, where they bring about a discharge of oxytocin, and this, circulating in the blood stream, eventually reaches and stimulates the mammary glands. The milk-ejection response thus involves pathways that are in part neural and in part hormonal, and it is therefore often described as a neuro-endocrine reflex.

7. *Frog Bladder Activity*, indicated by an increase in the permeability of the bladder of the frog *in vitro*, resulting in the movement of water through its wall. This also is an undoubted hormonal phenomenon, constituting one of several processes that maintain water balance in frogs; these we shall be referring to again later.

Distribution of the Hypothalamic Hormones in the Vertebrates

The combination of amino-acid analysis with these pharmacological tests has made it possible to investigate in broad terms the distribution of the hypothalamic polypeptides in the main groups of vertebrates, but in considering the results of this it must be emphasized that at present very few species have been examined; our generalizations, therefore, must be regarded as very tentative ones.

Within these limits, it can be said that oxytocic activity is present in the pituitary gland in fish, amphibians, reptiles, birds, and mammals, but not in lampreys. In birds and mammals, and perhaps also in reptiles, it is due to oxytocin, but this may not be true of amphibians, and there is certainly good evidence that both elasmobranchs and teleosts have developed one or more characteristic oxytocic polypeptides that differ from that substance. Thus the pharmacological spectrum of the oxytocin-like secretion of the pollack, hake, and carp is markedly different from that of synthetic oxytocin, and the name ichthyotocin has already been suggested for it, although its chemical composition has not yet been determined, and it certainly cannot be assumed that only one such polypeptide is produced by the teleosts.

The distribution of vasopressor-like activity is somewhat less complex than this, and it has been greatly clarified by a study of the water-balance responses of amphibians. These are exemplified in the so-called Brunn effect, a phenomenon (named after the investigator who first studied it in 1921), that is evoked when neural-lobe extracts of mammalian pituitaries are injected into frogs or toads kept submerged in water. The result of such injections is a great increase in the weight of the animals, amounting to as much as 20% during the succeeding 5–10 hours, and it is readily shown that this is a consequence of an increased uptake and retention of water.

There are good reasons for regarding the Brunn effect as being mediated by a hypothalamic hormone, and as being physiological rather than pharmacological, for not only is it evoked by extracts of amphibian pituitaries as well as of mammalian ones, but its importance in the normal lives of these animals is shown by its markedly adaptive character. Amphibians, by virtue of their highly permeable skin, are prone to desiccation, and are greatly dependent upon the moisture of their habitat. We may thus reasonably suppose that the hormone concerned, which we may call the water-balance hormone, facilitates the uptake of water and enables the animals to take immediate advantage of any source of moisture that they encounter. The ability to do this would be of the greatest value in those species that are farthest removed from regular supplies of water, and it is thus significant that the water-balance response is more marked in toads than in frogs, for the former are more completely terrestrial in their habitats than are the latter. Similarly, the neotenous urodele *Necturus*, a completely and permanently aquatic form, shows a response that is even less than that of frogs.

The interpretation of this response in terms of the known properties of vasopressin and oxytocin is complicated by the fact that it depends upon a group of physiological mechanisms that are not exactly paralleled in the higher vertebrates. One of these is the uptake of water through the wall of the bladder, a response dependent upon the increase in its permeability to which we have just referred. In addition, there is an increased passage of water into the body through the skin, a movement that is accompanied by an increase in the active transport of sodium. Further, there is a response of the kidney, shown in a marked antidiuresis. No doubt we may say that the water-balance hormone exerts its action by its influence on cell permeability, and that in so doing it shows some resemblance to vasopressin, the mammalian antidiuretic hormone. On the other hand, it acts upon certain tissues that are not involved in the response of mammals; the skin of the latter, for example, is impermeable, in complete contrast to that of amphibians, while the mammalian bladder is not influenced by the hormone.

These differences clearly raise some doubt whether or not the water-balance hormone of amphibians is identical with either arginine or lysine vasopressin, although our discussion of other hormones has certainly shown that comparable situations can be accounted for in terms of specialization of the target cells, with the hormone remaining unchanged. However, in this particular instance it has been realized for some time that the water-balance hormone of amphibians must differ from the mammalian hormones, for, although both oxytocin and the two vasopressins can produce some degree of water-balance response in frogs, their activity is far too small to account for the very high degree of activity that is actually found in extracts of the pituitary glands of the frogs themselves (Table 3, p. 125). In other words, the latter must contain a hormone that, as far as the water-balance response is concerned, is far more active than any of the known mammalian hypothalamic polypeptides.

The clue to the nature of this unknown hormone was obtained when, following the synthesis of oxytocin and the vasopressins, it proved possible to prepare various analogues which differed from the natural hormonal molecules in the substitution of one or other of their amino-acid residues.   One of these analogues is arginine vasotocin (Fig. 43), so called because it combines the ring of the oxytocin molecule with the side chain of arginine vasopressin, and this proved to have an extraordinarily high water-balance activity, as shown, for example, in its action in the frog bladder assay.   No

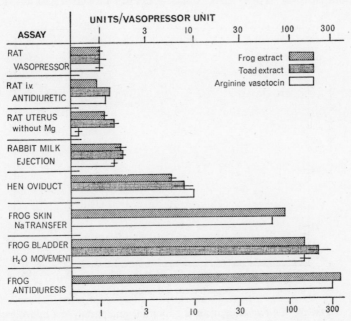

Fig. 46.   Relative activities of frog (*Rana catesbeiana*) and toad (*Bufo americanus*) neuro-intermediate lobe extracts and of arginine vasotocin, in selected biological assays.   From Sawyer, 1961, *Rec. Prog. Horm. Res.*, **17**, 437–465.

other analogue so far studied has more than 6% of its activity in this respect, and, as may be seen from Table 3, the potency of the mammalian hormones is even lower than this.

Such facts create a strong suspicion that arginine vasotocin may be the water-balance hormone of amphibians, and a study of the pharmacological spectrum of extracts of the posterior (i.e. neuro-intermediate) lobe of the pituitary of frogs and toads confirms this conclusion.   The relevant data are shown in Fig. 46, and they clearly reveal a close correspondence between the activities of the extracts and those of arginine vasotocin, except in the case of the rat uterus assay, in which the activity of the analogue is significantly lower than is that of the extracts.   This discrepancy can be satisfactorily accounted for, however, on the assumption that oxytocin is also present in the extracts, and there is, in fact, chromatographic evidence that this is indeed so.   It may be concluded, then, that the hypothalamus of frogs and toads secretes two hormones, arginine

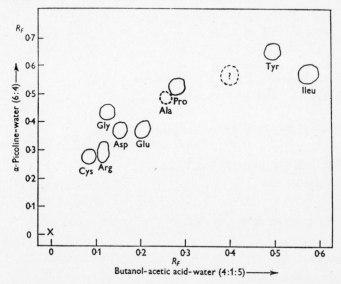

Fig. 47.   Drawing of a two-dimensional paper chromatogram of a hydrolysate of a sample of a highly purified hypothalamic polypeptide of the pollack, *Pollachius virens*.   The characteristic amino-acids of arginine vasotocin (cf. Fig. 43) are seen to be present, together with a faint spot corresponding to alanine and another that is probably due to a peptide fragment.   From Heller and Pickering, 1961, *J. Physiol.*, **155**, 98–114.

vasotocin, and oxytocin, and it may be pointed out that not the least remarkable feature of this finding is that we have here an example of a hormone that was first characterized as a synthetic laboratory product before its biological importance was appreciated; it would seem to be the only hormone that has so far been discovered in this way, although 11-ketosterone (p. 61) may prove to be another example.

This does not conclude the importance of arginine vasotocin

in vertebrate endocrinology, for a scrutiny of the pharmacological spectrum of neural-lobe extracts of the fowl shows that here, too, the data can be accounted for only on the assumption that the hormones present are the same as those in amphibians. The presence of arginine vasotocin in this species has been confirmed by the isolation of a peptide that has been shown to contain the amino-acids of that substance, and there is similar chromatographic evidence for its presence in the marine teleost *Pollachius virens*, the pollack (Fig. 47). It is thought to be present also in the cyclostomes, but has not so far been identified in elasmobranchs.

Evolution and the Polypeptide Hormones of the Hypothalamus

It is possible to construct a provisional scheme illustrating the evolutionary history of the polypeptides, although we must again emphasize that the evidence is still very incomplete, and that a more complex scheme may eventually prove to be necessary. At present, however, it appears that arginine vasotocin was probably the first of the known hormonal molecules to be secreted by the hypothalamus, and that it has remained an element of the vertebrate endocrine system from the cyclostomes up to and including the birds, but apparently excluding the elasmobranchs.

At an early stage oxytocin evidently appeared, and, as may be appreciated from Fig. 43, it could theoretically have been derived from arginine vasotocin by a single amino-acid substitution, the replacement of arginine by leucine at position 8. As we pointed out in our discussion of insulin, such a change might conceivably have been determined by a single mutation, but it would be a mistake to oversimplify this argument. For example, we have seen that there is evidence that the oxytocin-like hormone of teleosts is not identical with mammalian oxytocin, and it is even suspected that more than one polypeptide of this type may be present in that group. This fact, together with evidence that mammalian oxytocin is absent also from elasmobranchs, is by no means difficult to understand when it is remembered that both teleosts and elasmobranchs

are certainly not on the main line of ascent of the higher vertebrates. Each of the two groups can be regarded as a side-branch of
vertebrate evolution, and the development in them of characteristic
hypothalamic polypeptides may be seen as an expression of this
relationship at the molecular level. The lung-fish (and also the
coelacanth *Latimeria*) are very much closer to the main line, and
are of all living fish the ones that would seem most likely to secrete
oxytocin, particularly in view of the fact that the structure of the
pituitary of *Protopterus* resembles so very closely that of amphibians.

At some point in the history of mammals arginine vasotocin must
have been replaced by vasopressin, and here it is of great interest
that the latter hormone (in its arginine form) is thought to be
present in monotremes and marsupials, as well as in most of the
placental mammals. This suggests that the change must have
taken place in the reptilian ancestors of mammals (the therapsidan
reptiles), a suggestion that seems plausible enough when we consider the many mammalian features that are known from the fossil
record to have become established in those animals during Mesozoic
times. Indeed, in comparison with such major changes in organization as, for example, the development of homoiothermy and the
transformation of the bones of the jaw articulation into the auditory
ossicles, the emergence of arginine vasopressin seems a comparatively modest event. It, too, involves only one amino-acid substitution, in this case the replacement of *iso*leucine by phenylalanine at
position 3, and this, like the emergence of oxytocin, might well have
been effected by a single gene mutation.

No doubt much remains to be learned from further work in this
field, but we can already see in the hypothalamic polypeptide hormones a clear illustration of molecules that have certainly evolved
during the history of vertebrates. We have seen similar evidence,
although less clear-cut, in our review of other polypeptide hormones, and in at least one instance, that of the relationship between
corticotropin and the melanocyte-stimulating hormones, we have
found reason to suspect that such evolutionary changes may have
been the basis for the establishment of new hormonal functions.

Other examples were less clear in this respect, and we were left in doubt whether variations in protein hormones, or within the melanocyte-stimulating complex, have any relationship at all to new functional developments. It is the more important, therefore, to examine the hypothalamic polypeptides from this point of view, because their molecular evolution as so far elucidated has been comparatively simple, while the distribution of the variant forms is sufficiently well defined to be examined in relationship to the varying adaptational needs of the main vertebrate groups.

Two of the effects of the hypothalamic polypeptides stand out as being closely associated with important evolutionary developments in the history of vertebrates, these being the water-balance response of amphibians and the milk-ejection response of mammals. The former is directly correlated with the emergence of the terrestrial vertebrates, and with the failure of the amphibians to achieve complete emancipation from an aquatic habitat. We might, therefore, expect that an adaptation ensuring efficient utilization of supplies of water might be aided by the establishment of a new type of polypeptide molecule, but in fact this is clearly not so. On the contrary, in making use of arginine vasopressin the amphibians are taking advantage of the existence of a molecule that seems to have been established at least as far back as the cyclostomes.

In the same way the milk-ejection response is a characteristic property of the female placental mammal, directly correlated with the development of viviparity in the mammalian line, but the hormone that mediates the response is certainly not a new development, for oxytocin, on our present information, is already established in amphibians, and closely related molecules are present in fish. The significance of these latter molecules is not yet clear, and admittedly they may yet prove to be related in some way with particular requirements of aquatic vertebrates. The female placental, however, is clearly using in its milk-ejection response a hormone with an evolutionary record much longer than that of the mammals, or even of the amniote vertebrates.

Finally, the hen oviduct response deserves mention as an example of the opposite situation. Birds and mammals have had long and independent histories, after early divergence from a common ancestor, but ultimately the oviduct of birds must be regarded as homologous with the uterus of the mammals.   We might, therefore, look to find the contractions of these two organs being stimulated by the same hormone, but even this modest expectation proves to be unjustified, for oxytocin is the hormone primarily concerned in mammals, whereas arginine vasotocin is the one primarily involved in the oviduct response of the hen.   On the one hand, then, we find oxytocin, a hormone of ancient standing, being drawn into the regulation of a new need, while, on the other hand, two different hormones are shown to mediate two very similar reactions.   It is fair to add, however, that not too much weight should be placed on this last consideration, for, as we have already remarked, the response of the mammalian uterus to oxytocin may not be physiologically significant.   We may, therefore, be discussing here a reaction that is a by-product of the molecular structure of the hormone and that has not, in consequence, been expressly selected for the mediation of this particular response.

Chemical Transmitter Substances and the Hypophyseal Portal System

Our discussion has brought us to the point where we must admit that the diversity of the known effects of the hypothalamic polypeptide hormones cannot be accounted for solely in terms of their molecular evolution.   We are driven to suppose that here, just as with the hormones that we know to have retained a constancy of molecular structure, adaptation of the target cells and tissues has been a factor of the greatest importance in meeting the demand for new adaptations.   One aspect of this still remains to be mentioned, however, and that is the question of the function of the polypeptides when they first appeared in the cyclostomes and fish.   We have so far said nothing of this, for in fact very little is yet known; indeed, it has been suggested that they may have no action on peripheral tissues in these animals, for no responses comparable with those elicited in higher forms, such as the water-balance and antidiuretic responses, have yet been clearly identified.

It would, however, be unwise to set much store by this at such an early stage in the investigation of these hormones. Indeed, there is already a suggestion that hypothalamic polypeptides may play some part in the regulation of ionic balance, for neurohypophyseal extracts have been found to influence sodium transport in fish, a response that recalls the sodium movements evoked by arginine vasotocin in the skin of amphibians. Nevertheless, it is instructive to consider whether these polypeptides might not be related to activities of a nature quite different from those that we have so far considered, for the conclusions that emerge from this can retain their validity regardless of any other functions that may eventually prove to be mediated by these molecules.

In our reference to the structure of the pituitary gland we remarked on the association of the pars distalis of the adenohypophysis with the hypothalamus through the hypophyseal portal system, and on the growing belief that the regulation of the activity of the pars distalis by the central nervous system was effected by the passage of chemical transmitter substances from the hypothalamus through the portal blood vessels. While the evidence for this belief becomes increasingly more convincing, the nature of the transmitter substances remains in doubt. Nevertheless, there is much significance in the fact that some of the neurosecretory fibres from the hypothalamic centres end in close proximity to this portal system, instead of running on into the neurohypophysis like their fellows. This has led to the suggestion that they may be the source of these transmitter substances, which are visualized as being passed from the nerve endings into the blood vessels, to be carried by them into the capillary system of the pars distalis (cf. Fig. 14).

From this argument it is only a short step to the suggestion that the substances concerned may be hypothalamic polypeptides closely related to, or even identical with, the hormones that we have just discussed. The evidence supporting this suggestion is still meagre, although by no means wholly lacking. For example, the injection of small doses of vasopressin into the third ventricle of the brain of dogs has been found to evoke the release of corticotropin from the pars distalis, while other experiments have indicated that the transmitter substance normally concerned in this control may be a polypeptide closely related to vasopressin, although not quite identical with it.   Interesting evidence comes also from toads.   In these animals moulting is believed to be induced by the release of corticotropin, and it has been found that the injection of lysine vasopressin can also evoke moulting, a result that could be plausibly accounted for on the basis that this polypeptide promotes the release of corticotropin.   Finally, there are suggestions in some experiments that oxytocin may stimulate the release of prolactin from the pars distalis, but there is far from being agreement on this particular matter.

The point of view outlined above is an attractive one, but it is probably a mistake to link it too closely with the known hypothalamic hormones.   We have seen that the corresponding hormones of fish have not yet been fully characterized, and it may very well be that there are many other hypothalamic polypeptides still awaiting discovery.   In dealing with the relationship between corticotropin and the melanocyte-stimulating hormones, we saw that the facts suggested the possibility that there had been adaptive radiation at the molecular level, deriving from a particular synthetic capacity present in the adenohypophysis from a very early stage of its evolution.   A similar implication lies behind current speculations regarding the hypothalamic polypeptides, for it is perfectly possible that a fundamental capacity of the hypothalamus for the secretion of a particular type of polypeptide molecule has been turned to a number of ends under the influence of natural selection, leading, on the one hand, to the production of local transmitter substances and, on the other, to the production of circulating hormones.   For the present this remains no more than a possibility, but it is one that certainly merits further exploration.

The idea of the same molecule (or perhaps closely related ones) being able to function both locally and at a distance is not, of course, a new one, for adrenaline and noradrenaline provide examples of exactly this situation.   As far as the hypothalamic polypeptides are concerned, it could account for these hormones having only limited peripheral functions in cyclostomes and fish, for they may have evolved in the first instance primarily as local transmitters. At the same time, as we have pointed out above, the idea would remain valid even if further work disclosed that these hormones have wider peripheral functions in fish than have yet been discovered. In other words, the two modes of action, local and at a distance, may have evolved simultaneously, or the peripheral hormonal functions of these molecules may have developed after their initial establishment as local transmitter substances. Further than this we cannot even speculate, for we have no clue at all to account for the capacity of the hypothalamus to secrete such molecules. We have seen, of course, that its secretory activity may be regarded as an expression of the inherent secretory capacity of nerve cells, or of the ectoderm from which they are derived, but it is impossible to say why that activity should find expression in the production of this particular type of polypeptide molecule.

6 *Retrospect*

There is a passion for hunting something *deeply implanted in the human breast.*
Charles Dickens: *Oliver Twist*

IT will be helpful to end our discussion by bringing together the main conclusions that have emerged from it. We began by viewing endocrine systems as a manifestation of the fundamental need in living organisms for chemical co-ordination. We saw, too, that these systems are products of evolution, and that, in contrast to certain of the vitamins, they become in the course of their history as markedly characteristic of the biochemical organization of particular groups of animals as do the morphological features that have long constituted the basis of the classical approach to the analysis of animal relationships. In considering the implications of these facts our aims have been two-fold. We have explored the ways in which the various components of these systems might have arisen, and we have then looked to see how such systems, once established as characteristic features of a particular group, have been able to retain the flexibility needed to satisfy the changing adaptational requirements of that group during its history.

Evolution depends upon the natural selection of genetic mutations, and in an attempt to visualize how these may influence the development of endocrine systems we have had in mind three possible ways in which new features of organization may arise. Firstly, they may arise from structures that had initially no adaptive value of their own, but were merely by-products of other adaptations; secondly, they may arise as a result of the further intensification of the function of an already existing feature; thirdly, they may arise from changes in the function of such an existing feature. These three possibilities we have briefly reviewed at a morphological level of analysis, but we have been more particularly concerned with applying them to the analysis of the molecular structure of hormones. Now, in retrospect, we may well feel that the three possibilities become less obviously separable from each other, for morphological analysis, helpful enough in determining general trends, may seem over-simplified when we return to it after an exploration of the molecular field.

This is well illustrated by the history of the thyroid gland. At one level of analysis we certainly see it arising from a change of function in a previously existing organ, the endostyle, yet the primary function of that organ was, after all, secretion, so that the concentration of the thyroid gland upon thyroidal biosynthesis can also be viewed as an example of an intensification of a pre-existing function. Moreover, the initial appearance of the iodothyronines in the endostyle may possibly be attributable to the widespread occurrence in living organisms of the organic binding of iodine, a process that seems often to be a metabolic by-product of the presence of tyrosine and of the capacity of that amino-acid for readily combining with the halogens. At this level of analysis, then, we are invoking the first of our three possibilities, so that all three of these may well be factors in this particular evolutionary achievement.

We have seen, incidentally, that the history of the mode of establishment of thyroidal biosynthesis in the endostyle exemplifies a phenomenon that is also very well known at the morphological level of analysis. The endostyle did not become a thyroid gland as a consequence of a single major change at one particular stage of evolution. On the contrary, thyroidal biosynthesis seems to have crept in, so to speak, as a specialization of one limited area of the endostylar epithelium. Thus, in certain protochordates the endostyle provides a mixture of an ancient alimentary function and a new thyroidal one, and it thereby illustrates the 'mosaic' principle of evolution.

By contrast with the thyroid gland, morphological analysis has little to offer regarding the origin of those parts of the vertebrate endocrine system that secrete steroid hormones, except in so far as we can say that the tissues concerned arise from, or are closely associated with, the coelomic epithelium. We have, however, been able to learn a great deal more from molecular analysis. This has shown us that these hormones are products of metabolic pathways that are of virtually universal distribution in one form or another in living organisms, and that have provided a basis for adaptive radiation at the molecular level. Some of the hormonal steroid molecules of vertebrates must almost certainly have been in existence before the animals themselves had emerged, and in general it seems likely that the evolution of this group of hormones is a consequence of natural selection acting to favour the synthesis of those steroid molecules that proved to have some particular biological effectiveness. Some of them may initially have appeared as by-products of, or intermediate stages in, those pathways, and the incorporation of progesterone into the reproductive processes of mammals provides a particularly suggestive example of this possibility.

Evidently there is a wide range of potential variability in the metabolic pathways of the steroids, but despite this there seems to be a general constancy in the molecular structure of steroid hormones in all of the main classes of vertebrates. We have thus been driven to conclude that flexibility in adaptation has here been secured by modification of the target tissues. This solution of the problem may be supposed to ensure the maintenance of constancy in the fundamental relationships between the hormones and the cell processes that they are regulating, while allowing the expression of these processes to be modulated in response to changing adaptational needs.

The principle of the adaptive modification of target tissues seems to have been of widespread importance in the evolution of endocrine systems, for the steroid hormones are not the only ones exhibiting constancy of molecular structure. Other examples are the catechol hormones of the chromaffin tissue, and the hormones of the thyroid gland, all of which retain complete constancy of molecular structure throughout the whole vertebrate series. The wide range of response and sensitivity that is potentially available within the target tissues in such circumstances is well illustrated in the highly organized endocrine control of metamorphosis in amphibians.

We have found little information relevant to the origin of the adenohypophysis, although this organ is probably homologous with Hatschek's pit and the wheel organ of amphioxus, and perhaps also with part of the neural gland complex of the Tunicata, and with the preoral ciliated organ of the Enteropneusta. This implies its derivation from an organ that may initially have been both secretory and sensory, and it is just possible that that organ could have been concerned with the unification of the behaviour of members of the species through the agency of externally distributed transmitter substances or ectohormones (pheromones). We have been led by this thought to speculate that such an organ, initially concerned with external transmitter substances, might, by transformation of its function, come to develop a sensitivity to substances circulating within the body of the individual to which it belongs. Such might have been the origin of the reciprocal feed-back relationships of the adenohypophysis. The fact that its own secretions are complex polypeptides, proteins, or conjugated proteins, may perhaps be ascribed to further evolution of its earlier secretory products.

The pars intermedia of the adenohypophysis is involved in the regulation of colour change in lower vertebrates through its secretion of melanocyte-stimulating hormones. Some melanocyte-stimulating activity is also detectable in corticotropin, one of the hormones of the pars distalis, and we have seen that this is a consequence of the molecule of that hormone containing an amino-acid sequence that is found also in the melanocyte-stimulating hormones proper. This may in its turn reflect the origin of the pars intermedia and pars distalis from a common embryonic rudiment, and might be held to illustrate adaptive radiation at the molecular level, comparable with the well-known manifestations of this phenomenon at the morphological level.

This implies that there has been some natural selection of variants in molecular structure. Such variants are a common feature of protein and polypeptide hormones, and, when they involve single substitutions of amino-acid residues, they could well be the result of single gene mutations. Their significance is not always easy to understand, but variation of the more complex hormones may be part of the general phenomenon of the evolution of protein specificity, and it by no means necessarily involves any change in the mode of functioning of the hormonal molecule concerned. Indeed, it may well be that the biological activity of complex molecules resides in an active core that remains immune from such variation, because selection pressure would tend to maintain constancy of structure in that core. Variations could, however, become established in the remainder of the molecule without affecting its activity, although this part of the molecule may not necessarily be without any function at all.

We have found that recent advances in our understanding of the organization of endocrine systems have sometimes modified earlier interpretations, and this is particularly true of the neurohypophyseal region of the pituitary gland. It is now clear that the neural lobe is not a gland at all, but a neurohaemal organ, and that its evolution is a direct consequence of the development of neurosecretory centres in the hypothalamus. These centres, like the chromaffin tissue, can be regarded as products of an intensification and specialization of the fundamental secretory capacity of neurones, or of the ectoderm which gave rise to them, but this is a matter on which opinions are not agreed, and other interpretations are possible. The history of the neurohypophysis, and therefore that of the pituitary gland as a whole, seems to be closely associated with the functional link that is known to exist between the hypothalamus and the adenohypophysis, for some of its neurosecretory fibres are believed to regulate the release of melanocyte-stimulating hormones from the pars intermedia. There is also a belief that its polypeptide hormones, or other hypothalamic secretions similar to them, may regulate the activity of the pars distalis, for it is thought possible that these may act as chemical transmitter substances. The suggestion is that they are released into the hypophyseal portal system, and thereby constitute a link between the hypothalamus and the pars distalis, so that the latter is brought into relationship, through the central nervous system, with the external and internal environment.

There is still a considerable element of speculation in these views regarding the hypothalamic secretions, but it is certain that its polypeptide hormones show very clear-cut changes in molecular structure during vertebrate history. It is still uncertain how far these can be correlated with changes in modes of functioning of these hormones, but it is at least clear that important changes have taken place in the mode of life of vertebrates without any accompanying change in the molecular structure of these particular hormones. For example, the water-balance response of amphibians, directly linked with the difficulties of exploiting terrestrial life, are regulated by a hormone that is believed to be present in lampreys, and that may well have existed in vertebrates since the agnathan stage of their history. Moreover, the highly characteristic milk-ejection response of female mammals is mediated by a hypothalamic polypeptide hormone that is present throughout the tetrapods.

The distribution of available information has inevitably concentrated our attention mainly upon the vertebrates, but we have seen that the independent evolution of similar types of endocrine systems is very well shown by comparison of vertebrates with invertebrates, and we have discussed the problem of interpreting these comparisons in terms of homology and analogy. Neurosecretory cells are abundant in invertebrates, and even in annelid worms the beginnings of a cerebral neurohaemal organ can be identified. At a more advanced level of organization the X organ/sinus gland complex of crustaceans and the pars intercerebralis/corpora cardiaca complex of insects show remarkable parallelism with each other and with the hypothalamic system of vertebrates. Detailed comparison, however, reveals differences in organization and modes of functioning of the sort that are to be expected when a substantial element of analogy is involved.

On the whole, the available evidence, with all its present limitations, has made it possible for us to view the establishment of endocrine systems as part of a long-continued evolutionary process. This, we believe, has been achieved under the influence of natural selection, which is now recognized to have a remarkable capacity for building up essentially improbable systems by the long-term accumulation of small variations that, individually, may seem too insignificant to be of any importance at all. It seems likely that the results observed by us today could all have been achieved by the differential survival and selection of such small variations. In consequence, it seems unnecessary to postulate the sudden appearance of substantial novelties of structure or of biochemical organization, a phenomenon that is in any case no longer regarded as an acceptable basis for evolutionary change.

Almost all of the details of the course of events still remain to be filled in, however, and it is to be expected that future investigations will greatly clarify our understanding of the evolution of endocrine systems and of their hormones. For this reason many of the suggestions made here can be no more than tentative, and they must chiefly justify themselves by promoting present thought and future research. Hypotheses, like living organisms, must grow and evolve, and 'everything that is at all, must begin at some time'.

Further Reading

General

Anfinsen, B. 1959. *The Molecular Basis of Evolution.* New York: Wiley.

Barrington, E. J. W. 1962. 'Hormones and vertebrate evolution', *Experientia*, **18**, 201–210.

Barrington, E. J. W. 1963. *An Introduction to General and Comparative Endocrinology.* Oxford: Clarendon Press.

Gorbman, A. (ed.). 1959. *Comparative Endocrinology.* New York: Wiley.

Gorbman, A., and Bern, H. A. 1962. *A Textbook of Comparative Endocrinology.* New York: Wiley.

Takewaki, K. (ed.). 1962. *Progress in Comparative Endocrinology* (K. Takewaki, ed.). *Gen. comp. Endocrin., Supplement 1.*

Chapter 1

Bourne, G. H., and Kidder, G. W. (eds.). 1953. *Biochemistry and Physiology of Nutrition*, Vols. 1 & 2. New York: Academic Press.

Carlisle, D. B., and Knowles, F. 1959. *Endocrine Control in Crustaceans.* Cambridge: University Press.

Clark, R. B. 1961. 'The origin and formation of the heteronereis' *Biol. Rev.*, **36**, 199–236.

Durchon, M. 1962. 'Neurosecretion and hormonal control of reproduction in Annelida', in *Progress in Comparative Endocrinology* (K. Takewaki, ed.) (*see above*).

Mayr, E. 1960. 'The emergence of evolutionary novelties', in *Evolution after Darwin*, Vol. 1 (S. Tax, ed.). Chicago: University Press.

Scharrer, B. 1959. 'The role of neurosecretion in neuroendocrine integration', in *Comparative Endocrinology*, (A. Gorbman, ed.), pp. 134–148 (*see above*).

Wagner, R. P., and Mitchell, H. K. 1955. *Genetics and Metabolism.* New York: Wiley.

Welsh, J. H. 1961. 'Neurohumors and neurosecretion', in *The Physiology of Crustacea* (T. H. Waterman, ed.), Vol. 2, pp. 281–311. New York: Academic Press.

Wigglesworth, V. B. 1954. *The Physiology of Insect Metamorphosis.* Cambridge: University Press.

Willmer, E. N. 1960. *Cytology and Evolution.* London: Academic Press.

Chapter 2

Bergmann, W. 1962. 'Sterols: Their structure and distribution', in *Comparative Biochemistry* (M. Florkin and H. S. Mason, eds.), Vol. 3, Part A, pp. 103–162. New York: Academic Press.

Botticelli, C. R., Hisaw, F. L. (jr.), and Wotiz, H. H. 1961. 'Estrogens and progesterone in the sea urchin (*Strongylocentrotus franciscanus*) and Pecten (*Pecten hericius*)', *Proc. Soc. exp. Biol. Med.*, **106**, 887–889.

Chester Jones, I. 1957. *The Adrenal Cortex.* Cambridge: University Press.

Chester Jones, I., Phillips, J. G., and Bellamy, D. 1962. 'The adrenal cortex throughout the vertebrates', *Brit. med. Bull.*, **18**, 110–114.

Clark, F., and Grant, J. K. (eds.). *The Biosynthesis and Secretion of Adrenocortical Steroids* (*Biochem. Soc. Symposia*, **18**). Cambridge: University Press.

Dodd, J. M., and Goddard, C. K. 1961. 'Some effects of oestradiol benzoate on the reproductive ducts of the female dogfish *Scyliorhinus caniculus*', *Proc. zool. Soc. Lond.*, **137**, 325–331.

Fieser, L. F., and Fieser, M. 1959. *Steroids.* New York: Reinhold Publishing Co.

Gottfried, H., Hunt, S. V., Simpson, T. H., and Wright, R. S. 1962. 'Sex hormones in fish. The oestrogens of cod (*Gadus callarias*)', *J. Endocrin.*, **24**, 425–430.

Grant, J. K. 1962. 'Lipids: Steroid metabolism', in *Comparative Biochemistry* (M. Florkin and H. S. Mason, eds.), Vol. 3, Part A, pp. 163–203. New York: Academic Press.

Haslewood, G. A. D. 1962. 'Bile salts: Structure, distribution, and possible biological significance as a species characteristic', in *Comparative Biochemistry* (M. Florkin and H. S. Mason, eds.), Vol. 3, Part A, pp. 205–229. New York: Academic Press.

Klyne, W. 1957. *The Chemistry of Steroids.* London: Methuen.

Samuels, L. T. 1960. 'Metabolism of steroid hormones', in *Metabolic Pathways* (D. M. Greenberg ed.), Vol. 1, pp. 431–480. New York: Academic Press.

Wettstein, A. 1961. 'Biosynthèse des hormones steroïdes', *Experientia*, **17**, 329–344.

Chapter 3

Baggerman, B. (1960). 'Factors in the diadromous migrations of fish', *Symp. zool. Soc. Lond.*, **1**, 33–60.

Barrington, E. J. W. 1959. 'Some endocrinological aspects of the Protochordata', in *Comparative Endocrinology* (A. Gorbman, ed.) (*see above*).

Barrington, E. J. W. 1961. 'Metamorphic processes in fishes and lampreys', *Amer. Zool.*, **1**, 97–106.

de Beer, G. R. 1954. 'Archaeopteryx and evolution', *Adv. Sci.* No. 42.

Östlund, E. 1954. 'The distribution of catechol amines in lower animals and their effect on the heart', *Acta Physiol. Scand.*, **31**, Supplement *112*, 1–67.

Pitt-Rivers, R., and Tata, J. R. 1959. *The Thyroid Hormones*. London: Pergamon.

Roche, J. 1959. 'On some aspects of iodine biochemistry in marine animals', *Pubbl. Staz. zool. Napoli*, **31**, Supplement, 176–189.

Chapter 4

Dupont-Raabe, M. 1957. 'Les mécanismes de l'adaptation chromatique chez les Insectes', *Arch. Zool. exptl.*, **94**, 61–293.

Fontaine, M., and Fontaine, Y. A. 1962. 'Thyrotropic hormone (TSH) in lower vertebrates', in *Progress in Comparative Endocrinology* (K. Takewaki, ed.) (*see above*).

Geschwind, I. L. 1959. 'Species variation in protein and polypeptide hormones', in *Comparative Endocrinology* (A. Gorbman, ed.) (*see above*).

Harris, I. 1960. 'Chemistry of pituitary polypeptide hormones', *Brit. med. Bull.*, **16**, 183–188.

Li, C. H. 1961. 'Some aspects of the relationship of peptide structures to activity in pituitary hormones', *Vit. and Horm.*, **19**, 313–329.

Li, C. H. 1962. 'Some recent knowledge on comparative endocrinology of anterior pituitary, adrenocorticotropic, gonadotropic, and growth hormones', in *Progress in Comparative Endocrinology* (K. Takewaki, ed.) (*see above*).

Sanger, F. 1960. 'Chemistry of insulin', *Brit. med. Bull.*, **16**, 183–188.

Chapter 5

Harris, G. W. 1955. *Neural Control of the Pituitary Gland*. London: Arnold.

Heller, H. (ed.). 1963. 'Comparative aspects of neurohypophysial morphology and function', *Symp. zool. Soc. Lond.*, No. 9.

Jørgensen, C. Barker, and Larsen, L. O. 1960. 'Comparative aspects of hypothalamic–hypophyseal relationships', *Ergeb. Biol.*, **22**, 1–29.

Sawyer, W. H. 1961. 'Neurohypophysial hormones', *Pharmacol. Rev.*, **13**, 225–277.

Sawyer, W. H. 1961. 'Comparative physiology and pharmacology of the neurohypophysis', *Rec. Prog. Horm. Res.*, **17**, 437–465.

Index